How to Talk to Your Doctor

Getting the Answers and Care You Need

How
to
Talk
to
Your Doctor

Getting the Answers
and Care You Need

Patricia A. Agnew

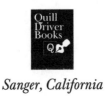

Quill
Driver
Books

Sanger, California

Published by Quill Driver Books/Word Dancer Press, Inc.
1254 Commerce Way
Sanger, California 93657
559-876-2170 • 1-800-497-4909 • FAX 559-876-2180
QuillDriverBooks.com
Info@QuillDriverBooks.com

Quill Driver Books' titles may be purchased in quantity at special discounts for educational, fund-raising, business, or promotional use. Please contact Special Markets, Quill Driver Books/Word Dancer Press, Inc. at the above address or at **1-800-497-4909**.

Quill Driver Books/Word Dancer Press, Inc. project cadre: Mary Ann Gardner, Doris Hall, Kenneth Lee, Stephen Blake Mettee, Andrea Wright

ISBN: 1-884956-54-8
Printed in the United States of America — fourth printing
QUILL DRIVER BOOKS and colophon are trademarks of Quill Driver Books/Word Dancer Press, Inc.

To order another copy of this book, please call
1-800-497-4909

Library of Congress Cataloging-in-Publication Data
Agnew, Patricia A., 1932-
How to talk to your doctor : getting the answers and care you need / by Patricia A. Agnew.
p. cm.
ISBN 1-884956-54-8
1. Physician and patient. 2. Communication in medicine. 3. Interpersonal communication. I. Title.
R727.3.A36 2006
610.69'6—dc22
2006017738

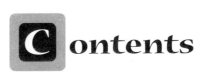

C ontents

Your Primary-Care Physician

If you are to be successful in communicating with your doctor, first you must have a doctor with whom to talk. The choice of your primary-care physician, the doctor you call first in case of illness or accident, is critical. You will talk to him more often than any other physician or surgeon involved in your health care.

You should develop a relationship of mutual trust with this doctor. You must feel that you can trust him with your health care, and he will need to trust you to follow his directions. It is imperative that he be open to questions and not bristle when you question his treatment or suggestions.

The choice of a primary-care physician is likely to be a top priority when you move to a new community or if your current doctor moves or retires. Remember that you are, it is hoped, choosing for the long term. Give adequate time and care to your choice. This is no time to close your eyes and stab the *Yellow Pages* with a pencil.

Establishing an enduring relationship with your primary doctor has its benefits. All of your basic records will be in one place. He will become familiar with you and your wishes. Together you will decide what is to be done when a health-care concern arises.

A bonus for choosing carefully, establishing a good relationship with a doctor, and staying with him is that a sort of bond grows between patient and doctor that makes the care of your health go more smoothly.

A quick note: Excellent doctors come in both genders. For simplicity and ease of reading, this book refers to doctors in the masculine.

Searching for a Doctor

A good choice for a primary-care physician is a family practice specialist, or what was once called a "general practitioner." You do not want someone "who only works from the belly button down," as a specialist once told an inquiring patient. Some patients prefer an internist for their primary care.

Depending on your age, another choice to consider is a specialist in geriatrics if one is available. It seems no one likes admitting to getting older, so you may be hesitant to consider a doctor who treats older patients; but someone who understands the problems and challenges of your age group is important.

When looking for a primary-care physician, be aware that discrimination against older patients is prevalent in the health-care system. The founder of the National Institute on Aging, a government agency dealing with all facets of aging, coined the term "ageism" thirty years ago to describe this kind of discrimination.

The older you are, the greater the chances are that your doctor will be younger than you. If, as you meet with the doctor for the first time, you sense that he is not really interested in you because of your age, don't waste time prolonging the interview.

Get recommendations

The recommendation of a friend—provided he or she has gone to the doctor you are considering for a period of time—is one way to find a primary-care physician. You and your friend probably like the same types of people, but in the matter of medical care, you may be quite different.

Ask what he likes about his doctor. Ask if he is satisfied with billing procedures and office waiting time; both are frequent problems for many people. Can your friend point out the doctor's strengths? Is the doctor a good listener? Is he skilled at explaining medical problems? Has your friend ever had to cancel an appointment at the last minute? Was he charged for it?

If you have a friend who is a nurse and has worked in your community, ask about the doctors she knows. Nurses see doctors in a different context and have had the opportunity to judge patients' reactions to doctors. Be aware of the relationship of the nurse to the doctor. Is it as an observer, an assistant, or an employee? Her relationship will affect her opinion.

Be aware of what the media is saying about doctors in your community. If a doctor has been involved in any questionable activity, you want to avoid him. On the other hand, a doctor who takes time to make an appearance on a local television show to educate viewers about one health concern or another and to offer information about diagnosis and treatment would appear to be a concerned physician.

If your community has a city magazine, it may publish information about doctors. *Phoenix Magazine* of Phoenix, Arizona, publishes an annual issue naming doctors in thirty-six specialties.

Community magazines may publish an annual health issue that is actually "information advertising." In my humble opinion, they should be labeled as such. These publications often have pictures of physicians and a list of their credentials and civic accomplishments. The listings may be useful for determining where a doctor went to school and took his residency, but they are usually paid for by the doctors and contain information that they provided, so take everything with a grain of salt.

If you are moving to a new community, ask the doctor you are leaving if he can recommend a doctor at your destination. He may be in touch with a former fellow student or know of someone through a professional association. This will give you a head start on finding a primary-care physician.

If you have just arrived in the community, ask the people you will be dealing with—real estate agents, garage mechanics, plumbers, and landlords. They all have a doctor. If you were to say to a stranger, "Tell me what happened the last time you went to the doctor," you would probably be glared at, but ask the same person, "Can you recommend a doctor? I need to find one," and you will open a floodgate of information.

Drop into a store that has a pharmacy, and ask the pharmacist for suggestions. Professional ethics may prevent her from recommending any particular doctor. But you can explain that you are new in town and ask her to give you some names without commenting on them. The chances are good that she'll volunteer additional information.

If you have a managed health-care insurance program, you will have a list of providers. Use that in your search. If you have located a doctor who interests you but is not on your insurance company's list, telephone his office and ask if he is now on. Things change.

Narrowing the search

Once you have names to work with and have begun checking the *Yellow Pages* for telephone numbers and office locations, you may notice that the doctors have different letters after their names. The letters M.D. are familiar. The letters D.O., which stand for Doctor of Osteopathy, may also appear after the name of a doctor in the same practice as an M.D.

Doctors of Osteopathy practice in all fifty states, the District of Columbia, and U.S. territories. The undergraduate training, medical school, internship, residency, and specialization of the D.O. are as lengthy and comprehensive as those of an M.D. According to the American Osteopathic Association (AOA), the difference is in philosophy: "With a strong emphasis on the interrelationship of the body's nerves, muscles, bones, and organs, doctors of osteopathic medicine, or D.O.'s, apply the philosophy of treating the whole person for the prevention, diagnosis, and treatment of illness, disease, and injury." Doctors of osteopathy also specialize, so specialists, as well as family practice physicians, are available. The Web site of the AOA, osteopathic.org, offers a wealth of information, plus up-to-date news and articles. The code of ethics is especially informative.

Considering that medicine has its roots in medicinal herbs gathered by cave dwellers, osteopathy is relatively new, having been founded by a physician only 130 years ago. It has been the author's experience in a community with a large number of D.O.'s , often in the same office with one or more M.D.'s, that you will have to read the credentials posted on the wall to tell the difference. If you are well past fifty, you may want to update what you know about osteopaths. Fifty years ago, in some states, licensing and attitudes were very different.

The doctor's gender may be important to you. Many women prefer a female physician. And many men prefer a male doctor. If you are choosing a doctor with your spouse, take him or her with you, but accept the fact that the same doctor may not suit you both.

The initial consultation

When you have resolved these choices to your satisfaction, your face-to-face selection process begins. Call a prospective doctor's office and ask the appointment secretary if the doctor is taking new patients. Explain that you are choosing a primary-care physician, give the reason if you wish, but don't feel you must. If the doctor is accepting new patients, tell him that you and your partner, if you are choosing together, would like to meet with him to discuss his becoming your doctor. Finding out what the doctor charges for such an appointment will give you an idea of what he charges for regular office calls.

In the same call, ask about insurance. Medicare may be your primary insurance, but not all doctors accept Medicare patients. If you have a supplemental insurance policy, mention it. There is no point in interviewing a doctor who does not accept your insurance.

Prepare for the appointment. Remember, time will be short. Many doctors schedule appointments at fifteen-minute intervals. You must get the information you need in that much time. If you are going with another person, both of you should write down questions and compare your lists.

If you have health concerns that require monitoring and control, but not necessarily the services of a specialist, ask how he treats those problems. Type 2 diabetes, high blood pressure, and obesity are examples of conditions that need control and monitoring but not necessarily the attention of a specialist. If there was something about your previous doctor that you would prefer not to see in this one, design a question to cover the issue. Be sure to take a notebook with your questions written in it, and take notes during the visit.

Arrive at the office a little early so you have time to observe the people in the waiting room. If you find yourself in a room full of pregnant women and wiggling, fussy toddlers, this doctor may not be the best choice for you. Is the waiting area over-full, indicating that the doctor is running behind on his appointments? It might be just that day, but make a note. Do you hear grumbling from the waiting patients? Listening may tell you whether this happens all the time or whether they are grousing because it is so unusual.

Are the people working in the office going about their tasks in a cheerful and quiet manner? If they seem harried and cross, there is a flaw in the operation. By eavesdropping you will be able to tell if the pa-

> 66 Prepare ahead for the appointment. Remember, time will be short. Many doctors schedule appointments at fifteen-minute intervals. You must get the information you need in that much time. 99

tients coming to the receptionist's window are complaining. The same goes for those staffers talking on the telephone. It is easy enough to tell if they are talking to an irate patient or consoling a regular.

Read the signs that are posted. Doctors tend to reinforce some of their rules by posting them in the waiting area. You may see some like these:

- If you need a prescription refill, please call the office before Friday.

- If your insurance requires a co-pay, it is expected at the time of service.

- Please sign in here.

- Please turn off your cell phone.

Not reading the signs wastes both your time and the doctor's time. Too many signs may indicate the doctor is too authoritarian.

Our society sets the doctor up as an expert. Television advertisements for new medications say, "Ask your doctor." Articles suggesting diets advise, "Always ask your doctor." Exercise gurus and advice columnists caution, "Talk to your doctor." He has been established as all-knowing in your subconscious before you walk into his office. That can make him intimidating without that intention on his part.

> 66 Writing down the questions you have and the information you wish to share with the doctor can keep you from forgetting an important point or burying the doctor in useless information. 99

Writing down the questions you have and the information you wish to share with the doctor can keep you from forgetting an important point or burying the doctor in useless information.

Your assessment will begin when he walks into the consulting room. Does he breeze in with a smile or come in as if the weight of the world rested squarely on his shoulders? As the interview progresses, be aware of your inner feelings about him as a person. Do you feel intimidated? Some feeling of intimidation is natural. If it is overwhelming, this may not be the doctor for you. The day will come when you will be lying flat on your back with little to no clothes on, and he will be standing, looking down on you. How will you feel under those circumstances? The paper costumes offered as a concession to your modesty do little to help.

Remember, this person is going to physically touch you—intimately. Do you think you will be comfortable with that? If you feel acutely uncomfortable with that eventuality, you may need to keep looking. How would you feel about discussing sensitive subjects with this person—sexual problems, family violence, incontinence, addiction, depression, or death?

Look for signs of compassion and interest—in his voice, his body language, and his facial expressions. Does he seem interested in you as a person? Does he make eye contact, or is he fiddling with his papers and looking everywhere except at you?

Choosing a doctor is about how he makes you feel. You won't be able to communicate with a physician who intimidates you, makes you uncomfortable, or seems not to care. Although your relationship with your doctor is a business arrangement and not a love match, the quality of care you receive will depend in part on your ability to relax in his presence.

If he asks for a personal medical background at this time, answer his questions; but don't waste your limited appointment time volunteering more than he asks for. If he is not the one you choose, it won't matter, and if he is, it will be collected later.

Do give him some information about your lifestyle. Are you a person who pursues a strict vegetarian diet, sky dives on weekends, and goes to Florida to wrestle alligators on your vacation? If you tell him and note an expression of shock on his face, you should look for a doctor who can follow up on a gator bite. If you prefer to read, golf, garden, and vacation at a five-star spa, let him know.

You may be able to use the time of this appointment more efficiently if you follow the example of Joy L. Holdread, a sculptor who owns Clay Objects Studio in Tucson, Arizona. She wrote a description of her lifestyle for both the doctor she chose as her primary-care physician and the heart specialist to whom he later referred her.

She felt that neither doctor was likely to know much about a clay artist's lifestyle. Since it involves lifting seventy-five pounds of clay at times, in addition to climbing ladders to arrange a show, and then spending long hours standing during public appearances, she wanted them to know. By handing them a printed page they could read in one minute, she saved the time of a conversation which might have gone like this:

> Doctor: "What do you do for a living?"
> Joy: "I'm an artist."
> Doctor, imagining watercolor paintings.: "What kind of artist?"
> Joy: "I work in clay."

Doctor: "Oh, I see."
(Although he probably doesn't.)

The doctor's approach to treatment will be determined by his background, training, and personality, just as your expectations are determined by your personality. If you are a patient who wants the doctor to make decisions for you, watch for signs that the doctor you are interviewing is the authoritative, take-charge type. The degree of trust that he inspires—even on first meeting—is very important. Will you feel secure putting your health care in his hands?

Being a responsible patient

This book is directed to the patient who wants to share in decisions involving his or her health care. For that person, the doctor needs to be open to questions and to be a good listener. Watch for this quality as you talk to him.

A doctor's approach to medical care can vary by region and by community. If you are moving from one part of the country to another, be aware that you may find different attitudes and approaches to treatment.

One difference in treatment pretty much cuts across all geographic lines. Here doctors tend to divide into two groups: those who are aggressive, pounce on a problem, order tests, and are determined to get to the bottom of the issue fast and the more conservative group that tends to take a wait-and-see attitude. (Studies have shown that, given time, perhaps as many as 70 percent of all ailments will go away on their own.)

You may be able to tell by the doctor's attitude and choice of words in the initial interview to which group he belongs. If you can't tell, ask. Your preferences will depend on your personality and how you feel about treatment. If you prefer to hand a good portion of the decision making over to the doctor, the aggressive approach may suit you better. You will have less participation in your treatment, but you will be relieved of some responsibility too. Or if you are the get-it-done-now type, you may want the doctor to do everything possible as quickly as possible. Of course, different symptoms require different approaches.

If you are more inclined to wait and see—and don't confuse this with procrastination, which can be dangerous—you may prefer a doctor who is more conservative. This doctor should be willing to discuss possibilities with you, as well as to outline a course of treatment should these possibilities develop, and to discuss a timeline with you.

Something that may not be at the top of your requirement list, which is still very important, is a doctor's sense of humor. Medical practice isn't stand-up comedy, but a little humor is usually a good thing. You will be more at home with a doctor who is on the same wavelength as you. This is where the generation gap can show up. Verbal expressions and situations that amuse you may go right over a younger person's head. The reverse is also true. At some point during your initial interview you may get a glimpse of what this doctor considers funny. Beware if it is something that you consider offensive or incomprehensible, because he is likely to respond the same way when you are his patient. And this may become irksome.

If your previous doctor had a habit that you did not like, address the issue. For example, perhaps your previous doctor had a physician assistant (PA) in his office, and you were frequently offered an appointment with this person instead of the doctor himself. Ask this doctor if he employs a physician's assistant and how the PA fits into the treatment program.

Business questions are important. Tell the doctor that you have questions about billing, payment, and insurance. Ask if you should inquire at the front desk about them or if he prefers to answer them. The staff member in charge of collection and billing may know more about those things than the doctor, and this may be the best person to direct such questions to.

You also want to know how to get in touch with the doctor outside of office hours or in case of an emergency. Will he respond, or will he expect you to go to a hospital emergency room?

Find out if prescriptions are written whenever you need them, or if the doctor has a schedule on which he writes them. Some doctors require several days' notice to renew a prescription; others do not answer requests for refills on Fridays, and so forth.

Retirement age is younger for all professions today. Judge the age of the doctor you are interviewing. Tell him you would like a long-term relationship with the doctor you choose. Ask if retirement or some other move that would preclude your being his patient is on the horizon for him. You don't want to come to the office next month and find a sign on the door that says, "Gone to Bali."

When the appointment ends, thank him and ask how he feels about accepting you as a patient. Although his willingness to talk with you implies that he was willing to accept a new patient, ask anyway. This doesn't mean you have made up your mind; it just clears the way. You will want time to think about this and to discuss it with your spouse or partner, if you brought a second person with you. Be sure to pay your bill on the way out.

If you have questions for his staff, stop at the desk and ask. You will want to know the basic unit of time that this doctor allows for an appointment and how long you may expect to wait for one. Ask about transferring your records. Make sure to get the address and the name of the person to whom they should be sent. The office may prefer to have you inform your previous doctor of the need for the records and then make the request themselves.

It is very important to know the hospital or hospitals where this doctor is able to practice. If your community has many hospitals and you prefer one over another, this may be a deciding factor in your choice. Hospital rating systems are available in communities with several hospitals.

When you are satisfied, thank the office staff and request a card with the doctor's name, address, and phone number. Keep it with the notebook you used for the consultation.

When you have all the answers you can get and you have interviewed as many doctors as you feel necessary, sit down with the information and begin checking credentials. If you use a computer, you will find it very easy to get basic information. A number of Web sites rate doctors. The American Medical Association offers a list of virtually every physician in the United States (ama-assn.org). Ratemds.com is a site where patients can rate their doctors. Here you will find doctors listed for both Canada and the United States. You can read the comments posted by the patients or even post one yourself about your own doctor.

Some Web sites charge for information, but it may well be worth the fee if you find the doctor you were considering has a reputation that equals Atilla the Hun's.

Other Health-Care Providers

Depending on your personal needs and preferences, you may choose another health-care professional as your primary health-care provider. The scope of practice of each of the following health-care professionals is prescribed by the laws of the state in which you live. You can find specific information by contacting the agency in your state that licenses them. A wealth of up-to-date information is also available on the Web sites of the respective professional organizations governing each of the professionals discussed below.

Nurse practitioner

A licensed nurse practitioner is a registered nurse with advanced education and training in a specialized area, such as family and adult health care, women's health/ob-gyn, geriatrics, pediatrics/neonatal, or occupational health care. The American Academy of Nurse Practitioners (AANP) in its role position statement states, "Nurse practitioners assess and manage both medical and nursing problems. Their practice emphasizes health promotion and maintenance, disease prevention, and the diagnosis and management of acute and chronic diseases. This includes taking histories, conducting physical examinations, supervising, performing and interpreting appropriate diagnostic and laboratory tests, prescription of pharmacological agents, treatments, and non-pharmacological therapies for the management of the conditions they diagnose. The nurse practitioner serves as a primary-care or specialty-care provider and as a consultant for individuals, families, and communities in a variety of ambulatory and inpatient settings."

Dianne Tobin, FNP-C, is an Arizona nurse practitioner. The letters after her name stand for Family Nurse Practitioner, and the *C* denotes board certification. This status is achieved by completing an NP program and passing a national board exam. NPs follow the rules and regulations of the state where they practice. "We're not trying to be doctors. We are health-care providers, but our approach is different, in rapport and time spent with the patient. We are experts in our field. We listen to the patient, talk with them, and make referrals when necessary. We know both the nursing model and the medical model of treatment and offer the best of both," Tobin says. "A big part of nursing has always been listening to the patients and taking time to find out what is troubling them."

Nurse practitioners continue this model in private practice. In fact, therapeutic listening and attention to the whole person are emphasized by the AANP. Consequently, you may receive more comfort from an NP than from a doctor working under the time constraints of today's doctors.

There are more than 100,000 nurse practitioners in the U.S. today. If you are looking for a health-care provider who will spend more time with you, consider a nurse practitioner. You may find a nurse practitioner practicing alone or in a physician's office. See the American Academy of Nurse Practitioners Web site at aanp.org.

Physician assistant

"A nurse practitioner is not to be confused with a physician assistant [PA]", Tobin explains. An NP may work in a doctor's office but a PA *must* work under a doctor's supervision and does not practice independently. Most PAs have at least a bachelor's degree. This is followed by specialized training in their chosen medical specialty. In order to be licensed by the state in which they practice they must pass the certification exam of the National Commission on Certification of Physician Assistants (NCCPA). You may meet a physician assistant working with a doctor or under a doctor's supervision but exercising autonomy in a broad range of services. PAs may conduct physical exams, diagnose and treat illnesses, and, in most states, write prescriptions. At this writing, only Mississippi does not have a licensing procedure in place for PAs. Information about PA certification and practice is available at the American Academy of Physician Assistants' Web site: aapa.org.

Doctors of chiropractic

The common designation of this health-care professional is chiropractor. A chiropractor is often consulted for aches and pains. However, according to the American Chiropractic Association (ACA), a chiropractor's scope is much broader: "Doctors of chiropractic are physicians who consider man as an integrated being and give special attention to the physiological and biochemical aspects, including structural, spinal, musculoskeletal, neurological, vascular, nutritional, emotional, and environmental relationships." That is a mouthful of long words, and your best translation would come from the chiropractor you plan to choose as a partner in your health care. As with any health-care professional, ask for an interview appointment before making your decision.

The ACA further states that chiropractic is a "drug free, nonsurgical science and, as such, does not include pharmaceuticals or incisive surgery." Additional information is available at the ACA Web site: amerchiro.org.

Doctors of chiropractic are licensed in all fifty states, the District of Columbia, and many U.S. territories. More information is offered on the Federation of Chiropractic Licensing Boards Web site, fclb.org. If you have trouble locating a doctor in this field, look under *C* in most telephone books. Doctors of chiropractic are not included among physicians and surgeons in the *Yellow Pages*.

Naturopathic and homeopathic physicians

As technology exploded in the twentieth century and was embraced by the medical profession, interest in naturopathic and homeopathic medicine declined. In recent years there has been a renewed interest in alternative medicine practitioners who employ herbs and other natural remedies rather than pharmaceuticals. Physicians in practice can be found in the telephone book or on the Internet. You can find a listing service at 1800Schedule.com or by calling 1-800-SCHEDULE. Also try the American Association of Naturopathic Physicians (AANP) at naturopathic.org or homeopathyhome.com. If you are consulting several health-care professionals, be sure to tell each of them that you are consulting the others. That way you can avoid conflicting treatments.

> 66 *In recent years there has been a renewed interest in alternative medicine practitioners who employ herbs and other natural remedies rather than pharmaceuticals.* 99

Concierge, retainer, or boutique medicine

A discussion about selecting a doctor would not be complete without a mention of a new facet of medical practice that has developed in recent years. Called *retainer*, *concierge*, or *boutique* medicine, it involves the payment of an annual membership fee in return for which the patient is accepted into the practice of a doctor who limits his patient load to a certain number of patients. These doctors see only eight or ten patients a day. According to MDVIP, a large company that accepts these fees on behalf of doctors, the patient is guaranteed quick appointments, twenty-four-hour access to the doctor, and ample appointment time. The company spokesman says the emphasis is on prevention.

According to MDVIP, the fee covers a comprehensive examination to determine the patient's health, after which the patient meets with the doctor to design a personalized health-care plan. Subsequent appointments are paid for by the patient's insurance or Medicare.

If money is not a consideration for you, and/or the doctor you choose has converted to a concierge practice, this may be an option to consider. Medicare and some insurers have expressed reservations about this practice, believing that it will discriminate against low-income patients.

Some doctors have converted on their own, without a consultant company, to avoid the hassle of too many patients and too little time. You may visit mdvip.com on the Web or contact MDVIP at 6001 Broken Sound Parkway NW, Suite 100, Boca Raton, Florida 33487. Or telephone them at 866-696-3847. An Internet search for "boutique medicine" will connect you with other services of the same type.

Rating the Primary-Care Provider

There is an immense amount of help for rating a doctor on the Internet. Start your search by typing in the name of your state, followed by *Medical Board*, followed by *MD* or *DO*, *nurse practitioner*, or *physician assistant*. This will likely take you to a site where you can enter the name of the person you wish to know more about.

Sites differ by state. Some list disciplinary actions, some do not. Some list the doctor's medical school, residency hospital, additional board credentials, and the doctor's medical license number. Disciplinary actions are usually listed by date as pending. At least one site tells you what the charge or complaint is against the health-care provider.

If you have difficulty finding your state medical board, you should know that not all states use that designation. Indiana, for example, uses "Health Professional Bureau." South Carolina has a Department of Labor, Licensing and Regulation. For help in this area try docboard.org, the Web site of the Association of Medical Board Executive Directors.

If you can't find what you need on the Internet, call your state government information line listed in your phone book.

You can find an ocean of information for free, but if you want someone to do the searching for you, there are sites that will get the information for you for a fee. There is one site that works like Amazon.com, giving you a shopping cart into which you drop your doctor's name plus the pieces of information you want about him. Then you check out with your credit card. Rated the best in a June 2004 survey by *Smart Money* magazine were DocInfo at docinfo.org and HealthPulse at choicetrust.com.

Since you will want to rate your doctor on how he makes you feel, as well as facts gathered about him, use the Doctor Rating Chart in the Patient's Tool Kit at the back of this book. It has space for your opinions as well as the facts.

Better Ready than Not

An appointment with your doctor is a vital key to your well being. You would not expect to impress a new customer in a business meeting without planning ahead. You would carefully prepare a presentation to bring about an outcome in your favor. You need to prepare for a medical appointment in the same way.

Maximizing Your Time with the Doctor

Preparation does not apply to sudden-onset problems, whose origin may be a mystery. You already know how to dial 911. For other appointments, preparing ahead will save you time, money and stress.

Preparation begins when you make your appointment

Various people may be assigned to the duty of appointment clerk in a doctor's office. Whoever is acting as appointment clerk will ask you what is wrong or why you wish to see the doctor. Some patients are offended by the suggestion that they discuss confidential health information with someone who may not even be a registered nurse. That person is not asking you to share intimate details of your problem, only generalities that will determine the amount of time the doctor will need to address your concerns. Give her an honest answer.

The basic time unit for an appointment is fifteen minutes, as we have already discussed. However, the appointment clerk usually has the power to allow for more time if you need it.

If you don't need an appointment as soon as you can get one—part of your preparation is to have considered your problem and decided how long it is feasible to wait for an appointment—be ready with your calendar when you call so you will know what days and times will suit you best. It is a waste of your time and the clerk's to wait until she offers you an appointment and then say, "I can't make it Wednesday at four-thirty." You will endear yourself to the appointment clerk, which can come in handy, if you are prepared to say something like, "I would like an appointment next week, but I need to avoid Tuesday and Thursday mornings."

The first person you talk to in preparing to talk to your doctor is yourself. Self-knowledge will save you time and money. A time-honored concept, *self-knowledge* is an ongoing process that you need to cultivate with regard to your well-being as you approach the age when more health problems are likely.

> **" The first person you talk to in preparing to talk to your doctor is yourself. "**

Pay attention to your body

No one wants to get old, so we tend to ignore that this is happening. But, while you want to avoid Chicken Little's "the-sky-is-falling" attitude with a minor symptom, you must consider that, if a problem persists for a couple of weeks, it may not be minor. A jabbing pain in your head that lasts for three seconds is probably not anything to worry about, but if it occurs again and again over a period of time, it needs attention.

This is not an invitation to hypochondria. It is not a suggestion that you ignore the fun in life in favor of spending your days writing down every creak, ache, and pain.

Later we are going to cover a written health history called a Personal Health Record that you should compile. It is something you should maintain on an ongoing basis. Label a file folder stored in a drawer or on the computer, and jot down the date and a one-line description of any recurring symptom that is out of the ordinary. If your feet are swollen after the long flight home from vacation, it may be expected. If they remain swollen for a week, you need attention.

Keep a record

You will need to keep notes and lists of questions. Choose your weapon—notebook, PDA, tape recorder. Use whatever method records a thought so that you don't lose information that might prove valuable when talking to your doctor.

At your appointment, you will waste time if you say to the doctor, "Oh, I don't know. Let me see, I think it was about a week ago. No, it was two, no, it was just after I came back from my vacation." Fifteen minutes doesn't allow for thinking aloud. You need specifics.

That is preparation rule number one: Be fully knowledgeable about the symptom you want to discuss with the doctor. How often does it occur? What time of day? What triggers it? Is there a pattern? Does it occur after exercise or after eating? Is there any one form of exercise that seems to trigger it? For example, does it happen when you are lifting weights or only when you are jogging? Does it stop when you stop?

Try to remember the first time you experienced it. This is important information. Was it when you were climbing the steps to the top of the observation tower on that day trip with your grandchildren? Check your calendar to find out how long ago that was. Memory isn't reliable. It may seem as if it were only yesterday, when actually the calendar tells you it has been six weeks. Write all this down.

Pinpoint the pain. Telling your doctor that you have a pain in your right leg isn't enough. Of course he's slightly better informed because you specified "right leg," but not much. Do the initial poking and prodding, stretching and flexing yourself. Is the pain in your groin or your hip joint? Is it in a calf muscle or centered in the knee? Pain can be elusive stuff. Put your finger where the pain is and move around. Were you right about the location, or is it really in a different spot? Does it hurt when you stop moving or only when you move in a certain direction? Does it hurt all the time?

Think of the time saved if you say to your doctor, "This muscle in my right calf pains me from this spot to this spot. It does not hurt when I am not moving, but when I change from a sitting position to a standing position it hurts. It doesn't hurt when I sit down again, but when I am walking it cramps."

That statement took fifteen seconds. Contrast it with this possible conversation:

"I have a pain in the muscle of my right leg."

"In your thigh?"

"No, right here."

"When does it hurt?"

"Well, it doesn't hurt when I'm sitting down, but when I get up, it hurts."

"Does it hurt when you walk?

That transfer of information takes the same amount of time, and you still haven't told the doctor that the leg doesn't hurt when you change from a standing to a sitting position and that it cramps when you walk.

If the problem is a sore spot that you have to poke around to find, take an eyebrow pencil and mark the spot with an "X." Do not use a felt-tip marker or ball point pen; they aren't good for you. Eyebrow pencils are made to draw on skin. Most men don't have an eyebrow pencil. Men, don't use your wife's thirty-five-dollar Hollywood-star-endorsed pencil. A no-brand cheapie at the discount store costs ninety-nine cents. Don't feel silly about this. Marking the spot is a well-accepted idea. A doctor about to perform a breast biopsy often has the patient mark herself with special pencil during the pre-op preparation if the lump he is seeking may be hard to locate.

Assemble your information. Write it down. You think you will remember, but you won't. There's a term called "white coat syndrome." This is where a patient's blood pressure rises simply from the stress of having it taken in a doctor's office. Well, this same white coat syndrome can affect your memory as well as your blood pressure.

Analyze the problem

Sometimes, an analysis of pain or discomfort may yield dividends. Consider "Jan's" experience.

> At a time when Jan's knees might have been expected to show some wear and tear, she was proud that she had never had any knee trouble. Then her left knee began to make her eyes water every time she got into her car. And she got into her car a lot. The first way she dealt with the problem was to brace herself for the pain and swear under her breath every time she slipped behind the wheel. The knee didn't hurt once she was seated or driving.
>
> Finally the pain became annoying enough that she consciously studied her movements. Exactly what did she do when she got into her car? She stepped up to the open door, facing the same direction as the car; she turned her body to the left, lifted her right foot— "Ouch." She looked— really looked—at her position. Jan was always in a hurry. As she turned her body, she simultaneously lifted her right foot, placing all the weight on her left foot. The left foot,

which should have pivoted slightly as she lowered her body into the seat, did not pivot under the full weight of her body and twisted at the knee instead. It had endured patiently for twenty years and was now complaining.

Jan's doctor didn't make any money from her knee problem, nor did the producers of anti-inflammatory drugs, or radiologists, nor did surgeons who do knee replacements. Jan now takes an extra split second to pivot slightly on both feet to allow normal bending of her knees to lower her body under the steering wheel, an action that takes six times as long to describe as to perform. She still has no knee pain.

A lifetime of those split seconds won't add up to the time needed for one appointment. Diagnosis, even with all the verbal information Jan could give her doctor, could have been elusive. It might not have been open to diagnosis until it was severe enough to require extensive treatment.

Especially for joint pains, it is beneficial to look closely at repetitive movements. Changing a habit can sometimes be as good as money in the bank and time on the meter.

Awareness of what you do and how you do it should be an ongoing part of your health plan and your action plan to improve communication with your doctor. This includes what you eat and drink and when you eat and drink it. If you notice that certain foods or beverages cause you difficulty, an accurate description of the problems will help you avoid a try-this and try-that approach, which consumes both time and money. If you suspect a dietary link, keep a list for a few days of foods, drinks, and the way you prepare them.

Realize that your body can change. Take a moment to think about even a small change that you may notice. A good question to ask yourself is, "What is different?" Ask it as it relates to lifestyle changes, as well as to how you feel. It's possible, for example, the seafood that you have enjoyed for years could suddenly land you in the emergency room with an uncomfortable or dangerous allergy. If several visits to a seafood restaurant—even over an extended length of time—have left you feeling queasy, it might be an allergy and not the quality of the food.

Paying attention to your body and keeping written track of symptoms in preparation for an appointment can help your doctor to make a diagnosis.

Handling Surprise Diagnoses

But what if you go to the doctor and receive a diagnosis that knocks your socks off? Maybe it's a life-threatening condition.

The possibility of a serious health problem can throw you into a tailspin and affect your ability to communicate. You may receive an incomplete or "maybe" diagnosis for which your doctor announces plans to order tests or exploratory surgery.

In the shock of the moment you might not know what questions to ask. You may find yourself walking out of the doctor's office, looking at a long-term sentence of procedures, holding prescriptions for a battery of tests you never heard of, without the information you really need to understand the issue.

You are likely to feel angry, scared, and betrayed. *Don't panic*. The truth is that very few patients perish from a delay of a week or even more. If they did, hospitals and specialists would perform tests and surgeries sooner than they do. If you were in danger, your doctor would have sent you from his office directly to the hospital.

Force yourself to go to the appointment clerk before you leave the office to make another appointment with the doctor several days in the future, when you have had a chance to prepare.

Then sit down, in the waiting room or in your car, with the notebook. (You did take your notebook, didn't you?) Write down everything you can remember that the doctor said. Keep writing until you can't remember anything more.

Go home and do what you emotionally need to do—pray, cry, swear, call in sick, clean your closet, or call your mother. These things are preparation, too. Then prepare for that talk with your doctor.

Become informed

Let us assume that the doctor has told you he suspects you have diabetes. This is a good example, because diabetes type 2 is on the rise in the general population, including those over fifty, and it is a scary diagnosis. It has long-term, serious implications. Get enough facts about this condition so that you can discuss it intelligently with your doctor. This ailment may be with you for a while—perhaps as long as you live. You will encounter complex information. Don't let it blow you away. Your goal is to obtain a basic understanding and to formulate the questions you

Why Did this Happen to Me?

The "why me" question is universal, and it is good to know if any of your past behavior has caused the condition so you can modify this behavior in the future. But, for many problems—especially for those of us over fifty—medical science still cannot provide answers to this question. You may feel victimized and betrayed by your body, but the culprit is likely to be the passing years. This is particularly distressing if you have done your best to take care of your health. You do not need to chastise yourself for getting older; it is out of your hands and the alternative is even less appealing.

will ask to get your doctor to fill in the blanks for you. Immediately begin a written list of questions.

There are two main resources for the information you need. One is the Internet, and the other is your local library. At the library, ask the reference librarian to show you how to find the information you need. Most library catalogs are now on line. If you have no computer knowledge, the librarian can help you with that too.

If you are computer savvy, the computer on your desk is your closest and most complete source of information. In fact, it is so complete that the avalanche of information flowing out of it may bury you, swivel chair and all. Chapter 5 is devoted to the importance of the Internet as a tool for gathering information that will sharpen your communication skills.

For right now, here are a few tips on using both sources of information to prepare for your appointment.

Use the library

In the library, ask the reference librarian to direct you to the medical reference books. Choose a book written for consumer use. The language will be easier to understand than that of a text written for the medical profession. A good example is the *Johns Hopkins Family Health Book*. The index is extensive and easy to use.

If you decide to move on to books that deal only with the problem you are researching, read the jacket information on the authors or editors. Medical doctors at teaching hospitals, scientific researchers at institutions whose names you have heard, and professors at major universities are preferred sources. If the author posed for the about-the-author photograph in a mask with a feathered rattle in his hand, perhaps you should look for another book.

Be sure to check the publication date. Medicine is a field where information goes out of date in a hurry. Open to the first page of text, not the introduction. If you encounter a lot of words that you do not understand, choose another book. There is not really a plot afoot to conceal information, but you might think so.

Take the time to skim a number of books while you are there, and check out the ones that seem the best.

Also examine the library's collection of magazines and other periodicals. Diabetes has got the attention of the media. You will find articles about it that were written for the general public, in language that is suitable for you to use in framing questions for your doctor. The *Guide to Periodical Literature* tells you what magazines have published articles on whatever subject you are researching, affording a quick check of back issues.

Use the computer

If you have just a little computer savvy, you will find the Internet a quicker information source. (Of course, a good reference librarian can help even the most dedicated Luddite.)

Information about most major ailments can be found at appropriate organizations' Web sites: the American Heart Association, the Ostomy Association, the American Cancer Society, the American Lung Association, the American Diabetes Association, etc.

Don't overwhelm yourself. Too much information can be daunting. Write down and absorb enough information so you can talk to your doctor, at least, about the major what-ifs. If you begin to feel confused or uncomfortable, take a break. Come back to it when you are fresh again. You might be surprised how what seemed incomprehensible at first makes sense after your brain has had a chance to subconsciously process the information.

Beware of sites that are chat rooms, where users share information about their experiences. Those are individual opinions about single cases that may lead you in the wrong direction at first. Later they may be just what you need, but for the first appointment, your doctor doesn't want to hear about the former lingerie model in Birmingham who had the same ailment.

Once you learn you have an affliction or disease, you will find your awareness of it will increase. A headline in the newspaper, a line on a magazine cover, a streamer on the television screen—anything about it will catch your attention. Be aware of all this; the speed with which new treatments and new medicines are developed sometimes outstrips a physician's ability to keep up. You may hear of it long before your doctor does. Make a note of the new information and ask your doctor about it.

As of this writing, this is the case with vitamin B_{12} deficiency. Vitamin B_{12} deficiency has been found to play a role in many health issues including Alzheimer's and other dementia, heart problems, some cancers, and infertility in young adults. It may even have a role in autism. For a number of reasons, this role is often overlooked by health-care professionals. A new book, *Could It Be B_{12}?: An Epidemic of Misdiagnoses* by Sally M. Pacholok, R.N., and Jeffrey J. Stuart, D.O., is helping raise the awareness of this phenomenon. [In the spirit of full disclosure, *Could It Be B_{12}?* is published by the publisher of this book.]

Gathering information can be addictive. Stop before you overdose. Your goal is not to become an expert—yet. When you have enough information to talk intelligently with your doctor, enough so that you feel more secure with the discussion and you feel you will be able to understand what he may say, go over your list of questions, adding and deleting as appropriate.

> 66 Take someone with you to the appointment. Your upper lip gets stiffer when someone is there to support you. Tell the person, 'I want you with me for moral support and to help listen and ask questions.' 99

By now you will have spent a lot of your valuable time in preparation. You should be proud of the job you have done. Don't yield to the temptation to try to impress your doctor. Let your calm approach and pertinent questions impress him. It is the best way to use the appointment time you spend with him. Your goal is to have enough knowledge so that you know if he is doing his job. Remember: Information is power. Your opinion will be more respected when you have good information.

Manage the fear factor

What if you are just plain scared? It can happen to anyone. Perhaps you have not had many illnesses in your life and therefore have had no need for tests and treatments. Maybe you will have to go to a specialist whom you do not know. Probably you are afraid of what you are going to find out. Maybe you are uneasy about the possibility of going to a hospital. So, what do you do when confronted with fear? Here are some strategies:

- Learn all you can. You will find that a good deal of the fear factor is removed if you have gained knowledge about your condition and its possibilities and probabilities. Knowledge is power. And knowledge will give you power to deal with your predicament.

- Examine other fears in your life and figure out how you managed them. Maybe you are afraid of heights, afraid of flying, or afraid of dogs. Will any of the strategies you have developed for coping with those fears work? (If it takes a couple of Bloody Marys to get you on a plane, you had better find another way to get to your appointment unafraid.)

- Talk to God. Prayer works well for those who believe in it, as does asking others to pray for you or with you. There have been several patient studies indicating that those who have someone praying for them do better than those who do not.

- Write down exactly why you are afraid. Fears set down in black and white lose their nebulous, monster-under-the-bed power. They become something you can confront, not something floating on the fringes of your mind making you anxious.

- Bag the guilt. Guilt can add to your fear. "Did I see the doctor soon enough? Should I have made this appointment months ago? Did I continue to take a medication that has come under suspicion? Is my problem my fault?" It is human nature to want to blame someone when something goes wrong. If you can't find anyone else, you'll blame yourself. Yes, you may have been doing something unhealthy. It seems one life style choice or another comes under fire every day. No one has a crystal ball. Even if you were doing something unhealthy, don't play the blame game. It is a waste of time and energy.

- Of course, quit any unhealthy behaviors and concentrate on what you can do to prepare for what may lie ahead and what you can do to get well.

- Confess your fears to someone you trust. Often, when you state your fears aloud, they sound minor and silly. Another person can help just by listening, but he or she may also be able to help you put them in perspective. Don't go to someone who isn't a good listener or plays the "I can top that" game. If you can find someone who has gone through the same experience, that person may be your best source of comfort.

Now that you are prepared, reward yourself. You have taken the first step toward solving your health problem. Fit an extra round of golf into your schedule. Go fishing. Rent your favorite old movies, and hide out for the afternoon and watch them. Call a friend for lunch. See if you can still fly a kite. Buy yourself something special.

Plan for the next appointment

Take someone with you to the appointment. Your upper lip gets stiffer when someone is there to support you. Tell the person, "I want you with me for moral support and to help listen and ask questions."

Do ask the doctor any questions you have, but be sensible.

You should now be ready to pick up your ever-present notebook and take command. The more you bring to this appointment, the more you will get from it.

You may feel that your appearance is not important when you go to the doctor. The major concern, of course, is your health. But how do you treat people when they look, as my mother used to say, "like they had been dusted out of hell with a soot bag"? You expect your doctor to be neatly dressed. You should be too. You may think he doesn't notice, but, trust me, he does.

As a woman, think about your makeup. The appearance of your skin is a good indication for the doctor as to what might be wrong. Some diseases cause your skin to appear yellow or jaundiced. If you are un-naturally pale or feeling feverish, don't conceal the evidence.

Prescription Card

In the Patient's Tool Kit section at the back of this book there is a form on which you can list your prescriptions and supplements and how often you take them. Photocopy the form, fill in the information, and keep it in your wallet. Keep another copy with your medical records. Be sure to update it when your medication changes.

3

In the Office

Before you can talk to the doctor, you have to get out of the waiting room. There are times when it seems as if that will never happen. What can you do about it?

The most practical approach is to have cleared twice the time in your schedule than you think it is going to take for your appointment. If you are taking time from work and the doctor is on time, you'll have extra minutes to do something more interesting or possibly get back to work earlier.

The Waiting Room

Use the time in the waiting room productively. Take a book. Take your laptop. Everyone knows about the outdated magazines in doctors' offices. Take the current issue of one you haven't read. After reading it, do the other patients a favor: Leave it for them. If you happen to be a writer, take a notebook and write down physical descriptions and scraps of conversation you may overhear. Who knows—the main character in your novel may be sitting across the room.

A good use of this time is to go over your list. Consider the example of "Charlie."

> Charlie went to the doctor with his list in hand. As he waited in the consulting room, he heard someone rap on the door of the next room and the doctor's voice saying, "Mrs. Moore, I can't possibly answer all the questions you have on this list. You'll have to shorten it." Charlie immediately pulled out his own list to see what he could leave out.

It can be hard to decide what to leave off your list. You can put your questions in order with the most important first, or you can try to consolidate them. Can you reframe a question to get one answer to two questions?

If you find that long waits are the norm in your doctor's office, there are several things you can do.

- Take the earliest appointment you can get. Doctors usually begin the day seeing patients on time. They run late as the day goes on.

- Ask the receptionist or the nurse if there is a day of the week that tends to have a lighter patient load.

- If you are geographically close to the doctor's office, which you may be in a small city, call the receptionist before you leave and ask if the doctor is running on time. If not, ask what time she suggests you come in.

Finally, don't take your cell phone. A waiting room is not the place for a phone conversation.

The Examination Room

With the nurse

Some of your time in the examination room will be spent talking to the nurse or other assistant. She will probably check your blood pressure and temperature, since both are good indicators of your general state of health at that moment. She will ask what medicine you are taking. Remember your list of medications from the Patient's Took Kit? Show it to her. It is even better if you have a copy you can give her.

This saves time. You won't have to spell out the names of the drugs or worry about mispronouncing them. Many drug names sound dangerously alike. While the information is likely on the chart or the computer screen in front of her, she needs to verify any changes. Tell her if you have stopped any of the medicines or added any kind of supplement since your last visit.

She will also ask you about your current visit. Give her the information as accurately and briefly as possible. She isn't invading your privacy. Her questions actually give you two advantages: First, they provide a dress rehearsal for what you will tell the doctor. Second, they will help you relax. She may ask you about any changes in your life. She's not being nosy. A parent moving in with you, the sudden responsibility of taking care of grandchildren, or any unexpected event can affect your physical health.

Alone

The interval between the time the nurse leaves the room and the doctor comes in may seem long. Don't waste it. Concentrate on remembering anything you might have forgotten, and check your list again. If you have missed anything, write it down.

Look around the exam room while you wait. Walk about. You don't have to huddle in the chair where the nurse parked you. The walls may be hung with large colored anatomy charts. Why not look at them? Most patients have a working knowledge of the human body even if it is just from high-school science class. You might even find a chart that deals with your problem. It's more productive than drumming your fingers, and it may ease any tension you are feeling.

With the doctor

At last, the moment you've been waiting for—the doctor knocks and comes through the door. *You* may think you are the most important patient the doctor is seeing today. *You* may think that he has your medical history in his head, at the ready. *Wrong*. Hopefully the doctor recognizes you as someone he has seen before, but that is all you can bank on. Unless you have a long history with this doctor, don't assume that he knows who you are, and don't assume that he knows why you are there. A friendly "Hello" and a smile are okay. No small talk. Remember, the meter's running. When he sits, you go to the business at hand even if he appears to be reading your file.

According to Dr. Wesley Johnson, a surgeon who was interviewed for this book, "Physicians are taught in training that a patient absorbs only 30 to 40 percent of what they hear—less if the news is grave or emotionally intense. They listen to one sentence and blank out."

You must not be guilty of half listening. You may be in pain, distracted, and worried. Even worse, you may have made a prejudgment about what is wrong with you. Your preparation should have made you more aware of possible issues, but the diagnosis is best left to the doctor. Listen and focus. Have your notebook ready. Ask your questions.

Remember to ask the most important question or bring up the most important point *first*.

"We look for the 'door knob' question," says Dr. Kelli Ward, a family practice physician. "That is when the person comes in for one thing and says he's doing great. And just when the doctor is leaving, the patient springs the real reason he came in."

Tell the doctor in your first sentence, "I'm here because I'm having intermittent pain in my lower right abdomen, but I had my appendix out when I was thirty-seven." You have told him why you are in his office, where the pain is, and have given him one clue as to what it is not. You can see the time advantage.

Every time you wait for him to pry the information from you, you use up valuable time.

Don't worry about how you state your information. He is the professional. He knows the long names for what you are describing, and he doesn't expect you to know them. If you describe a pain, try to relate it to a common human experience, one that he might have had. "It feels like pinching your finger in the car door, it hurts horribly. Then it kind of goes away." Or, "When it hits, I get really nauseated and have to lie down." Point out such things as whether you have headaches in addition to your abdominal pain or tenderness in your rib cage. Make your description something he can identify with.

Even if you have followed my suggestion, and have marked the exact location of a pain, he will likely still do what doctors call *palpation* and what patients call feeling around. He will probably cover an area that feels like the size of a beach ball in the general vicinity of your mark. Wait until he finds the spot and then yelp or say, "Right there."

Don't use idle conversation to cover your embarrassment if the doctor is examining an area that you consider intimate—some women are shy about having parts of their body examined, and most men hate a digital prostate exam; but unnecessary conversation distracts both of you from the goal of the procedure.

Don't ramble

When you start talking about your concerns, it is too easy to launch into unrelated things that happened to you five years ago or when you were twelve, or what you remember your uncle told you once about having a similar pain.

Your doctor will ask for your personal medical history and your family medical history if they are important to the diagnosis. If you suffer from some obscure ailment of which there are only a few thousand known cases, you should remind him. If he is your primary-care physician, that information should be in your chart. A one-sentence reminder will do. "Could this be related to the [unusual disorder] that I have?"

Don't bring up other pains or problems unless you think they are related to the reason for this visit. It is not the best use of your fifteen minutes, and the doctor may resent your taking additional time that may cause him to run behind on his schedule. If you had to wait overlong for your appointment, remember that the delay may have been caused by someone ahead of you taking more than the allotted time. Try not to be guilty of the same behavior.

Once he has completed his examination and discussed your concerns, he should be ready with some kind of answer for you. Now is the time to listen. Jot down key words as he talks. Some doctors love to draw pictures if they feel it will help you understand. Ask to keep the picture. If one of those charts we talked about earlier shows the locale of your complaint, ask the doctor to look at the chart with you. This might help you both to better communicate.

Medicine is not your profession, and in spite of your preparation he may use terms that are not clear. Ask for a definition of words you don't understand. If he gets carried away with the long words, you might try saying, "Doctor, you are too *sesquipedalian* (ses-kwee-pa-day'-lian)." It means given to using long words. You'll find out if he knows that long word, while indicating that you need him to use words you can understand.

The Next Steps in Your Treatment

The next step in your treatment may take any of a number of forms—a prescription for medicine, the recommendation of an activity or cessation of an activity, testing to refine a diagnosis, a change in diet, or even surgery.

Getting physical

If your doctor recommends an exercise program or physical therapy you will want to know what muscles or joints this regime is supposed to affect and what the desired outcome is.

An exercise done incorrectly may make matters worse. Ask the doctor if he can provide written instructions for exercises he has prescribed. Most doctors have printed materials available.

Diet

If your treatment involves a restricted diet, doctors are always well stocked with dietary lists of all kinds and will give them to you if you ask—gleefully, it seems. Plan to do additional research on dietary matters, since proper nutrition is quite important to good health.

Tests

As more tests are being developed for more illnesses, a frequent approach by your doctor is to order a test or tests. Some may be done in his office, but many are done at specialized testing locations. If the test is being done in his office, you will likely see him after it is done and can continue questioning him about it. If it is being done at another location, you will likely need another appointment with your doctor to discuss it. Either way, ask what he hopes to find out from the test.

Scientific names often sound much the same. For example, a friend once said to me, after she had seen her gynecologist, "I think she said I would need a *colonoscopy*—that doesn't seem right." The word was *colposcopy*, an inspection of the cervix, not colonoscopy, an inspection of the colon. Perhaps worse was the octogenarian who sent her friends into shock by telling them the doctor had prescribed Viagra for her. Actually it was Vicodin, a pain medication. Get it right. Write it down.

See Questions to Ask if Your Doctor Wants to Order Tests in the Patient's Tool Kit at the back of the book as well as chapter 7 for more information about tests. Additional details about most tests can be found on the Internet or at the library.

Treatment choices

If the doctor schedules a follow-up appointment to discuss the diagnosis and any proposed treatment, make another list of questions. Will the treatment be medication, therapy, surgery—or a combination? How long will it continue? Will you be taking medicine for the rest of your life? Does the doctor foresee a cure or only a treatment? Is there an outcome that your doctor can predict?

If treatment is complicated and there are alternatives, don't be stampeded into making a choice immediately, and don't panic. Ask for time to think it over. Many doctors will offer you this time. Do more research. Consider all alternatives. You might want to make another appointment simply to discuss the options with your doctor. Or you might want to ask for a second opinion from another doctor. You may wish to discuss options with a family member or a friend.

You need to plan how your chosen treatment will fit into your schedule and your lifestyle.

When you have made your decision you are ready to set up your treatment program. Have your schedule in hand and your next set of questions written down.

Your Expectations of Your Doctor

Defensive medicine

Medicine continues to change. Doctors are seeing more patients in less time. They suffer from an information overload of newly diagnosed ailments with scores of new treatments and medicines, and they are probably trying to have a life. As a patient, however, you have expectations as to how a doctor will act and react.

What do you do if your doctor's actions don't meet your expectations? Consider the case of "Susan."

> Susan had been referred to an oncologist, a cancer specialist, by her primary-care physician, who had not been able to find a reason for her symptoms, although they did not seem life threatening. Trusting the referring doctor, Susan made the appointment and appeared in the oncologist's office. He looked at her chart and blew his cork. He ranted on at great length about doctors who duck responsibility for a thorough investigation by referring patients to a specialist and expecting the specialist to order the tests and make the diagnosis.
>
> Having been told by a friend who had gone to this oncologist to expect a doctor who was very kind, but reserved and perhaps a bit shy, Susan was startled to say the least. Fortunately she was a mature and understanding woman who recognized someone's need to vent when she saw it. She understood that she was not the reason for

the tirade. She allowed the doctor to cool off and together
they were able to work out a satisfactory resolution.

It is possible that Susan's specialist was upset by a colleague who may have been practicing "defensive medicine," the action of ordering questionable tests or treatments or unnecessarily referring a patient to a specialist. These defensive maneuvers, driven by the rising number of malpractice suits, may also include a doctor's refusing to take high-risk patients. The encounter also gave Susan a new perspective on her primary-care physician. She soon changed doctors.

It sounds inane to say that doctors are human and have distinct personality traits, just like patients. But patients sometimes refuse to recognize this fact. It goes back to the god image with which patients have endowed doctors, the underlying and mistaken belief that the doctor knows everything and can fix anything. In the years before much medical information became general knowledge, as it now is, both doctors and patients subscribed to the idea of the doctor as a god, often with less than satisfactory results. Some vestiges still remain.

Miscommunication

When Charlie consulted a specialist he wasn't expecting God, but he found a characteristic more human than he was prepared for: a lack of communication. The case of Charlie and his doctor illustrates both the communication pitfalls a patient may encounter and how to improve one's own communication skills:

Charlie was hospitalized while on vacation with an
episode of congestive heart failure—his first. He was already
aware of his chronic obstructive pulmonary disease (COPD).

He was treated at a hospital by cardiologists and a
pulmonary specialist. When he returned home, he contacted
specialists in both fields, as he was directed by the hospital.

Only one pulmonary specialist was available in the
small city where he lived. The doctor was respected and
very busy. He reviewed the hospital records, ran a pul-
monary function test and oxygen usage test, and ordered
and read a chest x-ray.

He acknowledged the COPD, prescribed two inhal-
ers, and told Charlie, "You don't need to see me unless

you need to see me." Both Charlie and his wife heard him use those very words. The doctor did not specify a length of time for the use of the inhalers, and since this was Charlie's first experience with them, he should have asked.

Charlie used the inhalers until they were finished. He seemed to be doing well. He took the doctor at his word and didn't go back to him.

Two years later, Charlie's night breathing became so light that it alarmed his wife. They made an appointment with the pulmonologist.

At the appointment, the doctor's first words were, "How long has it been since I've seen you?" meaning where have you been?

Both Charlie and his wife repeated the doctor's words, "You don't need to see me unless you need to see me." Clearly it had been a misstatement, because the doctor had written on Charlie's chart, "Appointment in six to eight weeks."

With 20/20 hindsight it is apparent that Charlie should have ignored the doctor's flippant comment and asked, "Do I need another appointment?"

"If you had continued taking the medicines I prescribed, you'd probably be in better shape," the doctor commented. However, as Charlie pointed out, he had not given directions for continued use.

Both the doctor and Charlie agreed that there had been a misunderstanding. Fortunately there were no tragic consequences.

Charlie finds this doctor personable. His professional knowledge has not been called into question. He is extremely skillful at explaining complicated medical concepts in understandable terms. Besides, he's the only game in town, and Charlie would be forced to travel a long distance to find another doctor.

Because of his experience with this doctor, Charlie is more alert to signs of miscommunication. By being aware of good communications himself, Charlie believes he can overcome a doctor's tendency to not communicate well.

Doctors are human, and it is possible to encounter one who has

It's a Big Job

Do you expect your doctor to know everything? When you do not receive an instant and accurate diagnosis, remember that the list of ailments that a family practice physician might expect to encounter runs to a thousand or more pages. A similar list for an ophthalmologist is only three pages.

trouble communicating. But there are times when it is not possible or desirable to find another doctor. Perhaps you like yours a lot, preferring his compassionate attitude and professional ability to such a degree that you don't mind his lack of communication skills. In any case, you, like Charlie, can develop communication tactics that succeed.

Tactlessness

What can you do if your doctor's tactlessness offends you? You can change doctors about every third visit, or you can follow the example of "Catherine."

> *Catherine suffers from unrelenting back pain caused by scoliosis that was not treated in childhood, severe arthritis, and seventy-five birthdays. She went to her husband's doctor in the hope that he could give her some relief. At her first visit, he listened to her complaint and then said, "Get off your backside and do something active."*
>
> *Of course, he could not tell by looking that Catherine was very active in her church, continued a several-decades-long service with the Girl Scouts of America, was caring for a disabled relative, and had that very year embroidered, pieced, and given away twelve quilts. Needless to say, his comment was not well received. However, Catherine's husband and the doctor had good rapport. Catherine gave him another chance, and they eventually reached a comfortable understanding.*

4

Your Doctor's Staff

Who are all the people buzzing around in your doctor's office and what do they do? Each doctor organizes his office a little differently, but following are some of the staff members you might meet. If you learn who they are and what they do, you won't need to spend any of your precious appointment time asking the doctor questions that a staff member can better answer.

Locating Staff

The front office

You will hear the terms *back office* and *front office* used. In the front office you'll find the receptionist. In an office where several doctors practice, there may be more than one receptionist. After your first visit you will know which one signs in your doctor's patients. It is the receptionist's job to welcome you and have you sign in on the ever-present clipboard.

If you are a Medicare patient, the receptionist may also ask you to sign a waiver which explains that if Medicare does not pay for today's service, you may opt not to have it or to pay the charges yourself. If there is a procedure or test involved that you are not familiar with, you may ask her for the estimated cost. If she does not know, she will find another staff member who can answer your question.

Checkout receptionists are also front office personnel. They see you before you leave and take the sheet that the doctor has given you listing the procedures performed with their code numbers. If you are not given a copy, you might want to ask for one. Printed on the sheet are up to a hundred different procedures, with code numbers for the procedure and code numbers for the fee charged. Your doctor will circle the ones that match what he did during your appointment. The coded procedures are specific to the doctor. Different procedures will appear on a sheet for a family doctor than for a surgeon or other specialist. The doctor probably delegates the billing process.

If a payment is due, the checkout receptionist will collect it. If your doctor is one of the few who still sends bills, the receptionist will tell you. She may write the day's charges on the sheet you take with you.

Some offices may have a supervisor who oversees the front office personnel. Ask if your doctor has one and learn her name. If you have a paperwork problem, start with her. She'll be quick to pass you along if the problem is outside of her jurisdiction.

The back office

Your doctor's nurse may be a familiar face, since she works as a part of the doctor's team in the back office, assisting him with patients. In a large practice, each doctor will have his own nurse. Use her name when you greet her or talk with her. The nurse is an important link in your connection to the doctor.

She can often answer questions for you such as, "Should I stop medicine A before beginning medicine B?" If she is unable to answer your question, or if you don't have faith in her to answer the question completely or accurately, ask that she check with the doctor and get back to you.

She can ask him your question between consultations and relay the answer to you. This is the best and quickest method for questions of a nonemergency nature. If you are asking for the doctor to call you, find out from the nurse what time of day he returns his telephone calls. Try to be close to your telephone, and keep your line clear at that time.

The appointment clerk may be invisible to you, but she is critical to the smooth operation of the office. If you call to change an appointment or to ask for more time at your appointment because something new has come up, address her by name. If you are asking for more time, have your personal calendar at hand, because you may need to take a different day and time altogether. She is also the person to ask if you may be put on a waiting list, ready to come in on a moment's notice if the doctor has a cancellation. (If you have established a good rapport with your primary-care physician, the appointment clerk will usually do everything possible to "work you in," warning you that you may have to wait.)

Another usually invisible staff member, but one you want to get to know by name, is the billing person. There may be more than one, and it is possible that your doctor outsources his billing. But find a person in that department to whom you can address any questions you have about billing and its related subject, insurance.

A billing problem might have been caused by using the wrong code for a procedure, and a quick solution is more likely when you work with the person who has those codes at his or her fingertips. In some cases, if your insurance has been slow in paying and your doctor has his lab work done away from his office, you may receive a bill from a laboratory you have never heard of—call your doctor's billing department and ask if they can tell you what it is for. Have handy any insurance reports that you have received relating to the visit. Sometimes you receive a bill because your secondary insurance has not yet paid. The billing secretary will be able to tell you where it came from and why. Then call the billing party. Read the fine print on the bill. There is often a different number for billing questions than for office service.

A business office

Your doctor's office is a business, and it should be run by his staff in a businesslike fashion.

Is your file readily available so that your doctor can put his hands on the document he needs immediately upon beginning your consultation? Does your doctor's office call you twenty-four hours ahead to remind you of an appointment, on Friday if the appointment is Monday? Were you given a card to remind you of your appointment when you made it at the office?

If you must change an appointment, is the appointment secretary able to find your name on the schedule quickly? Are you reminded that your annual physical is approaching, assuming your doctor gives annual physicals? If you encounter a new staff member who is just beginning, does the person who is training her inform you, so that you can be a help rather than a hindrance? Is there visible tension between staffers? These are things to watch for. If a doctor puts up with a sloppily run office, his attitude toward diagnosis and treatment might bear extra scrutiny.

Relating to Staff

Patient-staff relations

Treat the staff members in your doctor's office as if they were important—they are. They have a good deal of control over how smoothly your relationship with the doctor proceeds. If he hears them groan when they find you on the other end of the phone line or coming through the door, how do you think he will treat you? Don't bad mouth a member of the staff to the doctor. He hired them, and he wants to think he made the right choice.

If you have a complaint, by all means, don't smother it, but don't strike when you're angry. Give yourself time to cool off—even if you don't want to. Take the matter first to the office manager, if there is one, and then to the doctor. When complaining, use proper channels. You'll get better results.

Gifts

Gifts are a matter of personal choice on the patient's part. I know a woman who is proficient in needlework and another who is an Avon lady. They have kept the female staff members in their respective doctors' offices in potholders and beauty products for years. These two patients never seem to want for free samples of medications and have no trouble getting a message to the doctor.

In one office, I have noted that there are usually some tempting snacks or a box of doughnuts sitting on the table in the lunchroom. Sometimes you can smell gourmet coffee. Let your conscience be your guide. Avoid liquor and cigars. Holiday time is when everyone remembers, anyway, so pick an ordinary day and brighten it for the staff.

5

The Internet: Your Ally in Gathering Information

You may not care about the Internet when your throat hurts, but it is a stellar tool to equip you with information for talking to your doctor.

Correctly organized, computer research saves you time. It is like having a limitless medical encyclopedia at your fingertips. Knowing how to use it is one of the best things you can do toward taking charge of your health.

Internet usage is increasing among all ages, particularly those over fifty. If you are not yet a fan of the Internet; or worse yet, if you have computer phobia, make yourself a promise to get to know and use the Internet as an ally instead of an enemy.

If you don't have a computer in your home, consider going to your local library. Most have computers that you may use without charge and often have someone to help you learn how to use them. A local college or adult school may offer computer classes.

Health is big business, and every facet of the industry uses the Internet to inform, advertise, persuade, and, if you are not careful, confuse you when you are looking for information. No matter if it is a company selling a product to enhance your health, a firm researching and marketing a new medicine, a university pitching for research funds, or a doctor with a newly developed surgical technique, there is likely a Web site for it.

Select any health problem and the Internet will offer you reams of information about it: causes, treatments, prognoses, the latest research breakthroughs, even names of specialists and specializing hospitals.

In chat rooms you can communicate with sufferers or caregivers willing to share their insights, which can come only from personal experience. Message boards offer you the opportunity to put your question to a host of people who may have already tackled and solved a problem that is troubling you. Stories abound about patients or caregivers who have done research on the Internet and found new, successful treatments.

Patients in the twenty to forty age bracket ask their doctors lots of questions, while those over sixty ask almost no questions. Could this be because the younger group, which is known to be computer savvy, has more information? If you're over fifty and have not yet availed yourself of this resource—it's time.

Search Engines

There are a number of Internet search engines. A search engine is a Web site that searches the Internet for other Web sites. At the time of this writing, Google was the overwhelming favorite search engine. Yahoo!, Ask Jeeves, and Dogpile.com are other choices. None charge for their services. They derive their revenue from advertising and for placing Web sites higher up in the list of sites shown on your screen when you do a search.

Different search engines work in slightly different ways, so one may locate Web sites another misses. If you feel that one search engine is weak, experiment with others. With important searches, use more than one.

Try this: Choose a disease in which you have an interest—let's use *lung disease* as an example. Enter *lung disease* into the appropriate place on the search engine's web page and click "search." You will get millions of "hits," or listings. When I did this, one search engine returned more than six million listings. This is because this search engine pulled up every reference containing the word *lung* or the word *disease*. The listings included everything from drug company specifications on certain medicines used to treat myriad lung diseases to a news bulletin about jewelry workers in China dying of lung disease.

This illustrates why it is important to narrow your search. With most search engines, you can limit your search by entering quotation marks before and after a term. For instance, *"lung disease"* would only return hits that include both words together.

Let's say you don't want information on all kinds of lung disease, but only on the type known as chronic obstructive pulmonary disease. Enter COPD, the acronym for the disease, and the number of hits drops to just below two million. It may be that the top ten or twenty sites listed have the information you want, or you may wish to refine your search further. My typing in "COPD chat room" reduced the hits to 7,000. "COPD acuncture" produced 296 hits. If I were looking for an acupuncturist in Miami, "COPD acupuncture Miami" would have further reduced the number of hits and possibly led me to such a specialist.

Each listing will include the site's name, web address, and explanatory lines. Reading the explanation will help you find the sites you want to visit.

Oops!

What? You hit the wrong key and don't know what to do? Hit the X in the upper right corner of the screen and keep hitting it until you are all the way out. Then start over.

Selecting Sites to Visit

As you can imagine, not all sites are equal. Since anyone can set up a Web site, be wary. Not all offer accurate or trustworthy information.

United States government and major university sites often offer up-to-date and reliable medical information. United States government sites can usually be identified by ".gov" appearing as part of their web address. The web address for the National Institutes of Health is nih.gov. Universities often have ".edu" as part of their web site address. The Northwestern University Center for Clinical Research's web address is medschool.northwestern.edu/nccr.

Nearly every disorder or disease has at least one organization devoted to informing sufferers, their families, and the general public about the disease. Their agendas, of course, include fund raising to find cures, but the information they offer is often useful. They are usually identified as the National Association of... or the American Foundation for..., or the American Institute of.... Often their web addresses include the designation ".org."

Medical publications such as *The New England Journal of Medicine*, *The Journal of the American Medical Association*, and *Lancet*, the British equivalent of *JAMA*, post articles or allow access to their publications online. Some of these require a paid subscription; some ask you to register; some are available only to health-care professionals. Articles from newspapers and other print media are often posted as well. By accessing major newspapers or using your favorite news site you can follow breaking news on the subject you are interested in on a daily basis.

Information from companies that produce or market medications or devices designed to treat or alleviate symptoms of a particular disease can be found on the Web.

In addition, there will be Web sites discussing how a disease is affected by environment, occupation, age, and gender. Some sites will examine the impact of certain medications on the disease. Some will discuss experimental or futuristic treatments. All of this information may be useful to you at some point in your treatment.

The Internet is not static. Information in a book does not change unless the book is rewritten and republished. Web sites change frequently. In fact, part of their usefulness is that they do change. Look for sites that have been recently updated or that are updated frequently.

The media offer sources

Sometimes a news story in the print media will catch your eye. Such a story may not give you all the information you would like to have. Many reporters now include a web address as part of the story so you can find out more on the Internet. Check the dateline—that is, the place the story originated—San Jose, CA, or Baltimore, MD, for example. The Internet can give you a list of the newspapers in that city, and you can go to their Web sites for the full story. It may include statistics and sidebars that were not reprinted in the publication you are reading. The writer of the story may tell you that this information came from another source. You can check the source's Web sites for the full story.

Searching "medical news" with any search engine will give you access to the current news stories about medicine. Google, in its cache of medical news sites, lists how many hours ago they were posted. If you happen to catch a thirty-second sound bite or streaming line on television about medical news that triggers your interest, try searching "medical news" to learn more.

Magazine articles may give a Web site you can visit or a book from which the article's information was culled. You may find the book excerpted on the author's Web site or on Amazon.com.

Check news stories about revolutionary new treatments when the treatment is due to be available. You don't want to waste research time or your appointment time asking your doctor about a treatment that won't be available for five years.

It's Called "Surfing the Web"

Surfing is a good term for plunging into this ocean of information, because just as pounding surf can drown the unwary, so you can drown in details doing Internet research on your personal health problem. The most effective way to use the Internet is to seek your information in stages. You are doing this for your health. Nothing could be of more importance to you. You'll want to know everything, but you will find it easy to get drawn into more and more detail. If you are an experienced Net surfer, you already know this. There is such a thing as information overload.

Avoid researching symptoms

Don't research symptoms. Looking up information on symptoms will give you too many possibilities related to too many ailments. Plugging in *headaches*, *muscle weakness*, or *foot pain*, for example, will give you hits on more diseases than you knew existed. This is useless. And it may lead you down a wrong path. In the matter of health information, don't be seduced. Once your doctor has given you a diagnosis, you can start to put the power of the Internet to work for you. This is your health. Nothing could be of more importance to you.

Take a class

Receiving computer instruction in a class is not always easy. There can be a lot of "Hurry up and wait," as class members struggle with new concepts. You may prefer to get a personal tutor. Check the classified ads, ask at the local high school or college if there is a student available for tutoring, or ask a grandchild or a friend. After one session you will know if the person is a teacher or not. Many people who are computer experts cannot teach. They know too much and they move too fast. If their fingers are a blur on the keyboard and what appears on the screen looks like a streaming movie teaser, you will be discouraged and give up. The best teacher puts you at the keyboard and walks you patiently through the process. You might also check health fairs in your area. Some offer sessions on how to search the Internet for health information.

You want to find information on the Internet, keep track of it for future reference, and print it if you want a hard copy. Ask your tutor to show you how to do these things.

Starting your research

Now you are ready to go after new information. Not every appointment with the doctor requires research. The sore throat we mentioned earlier is not something you are going to learn a lot about by keying *sore throat* into your search engine. But suppose that your doctor has indicated that you have a problem with your prostate? That's not an uncommon ailment for men over fifty. He will undoubtedly have treatments or further testing to suggest. However, there won't be time for him to give you a detailed explanation—twenty minutes and you are out the door, with a problem you didn't know you had.

Remember, you are not going to panic. You are going to give yourself a few days to investigate and then schedule the tests. Even if it is hard to wait, you will want to know more before you undergo the procedure. If all you really know about this ailment is what you have picked up in the locker room at the health club, it's time to dip your toe into Internet waters even if you are not yet ready to surf.

A good starting point is the Web site of the National Institutes of Health, an agency of the U.S. Department of Health and Human Services. It is a source of information about diseases, tests, surgical procedures, and clinical trials. If you do not have a favorite search engine, try Google. The results it gives are quite easy to understand.

Let's say you wanted information about prostate disease. Go to Google and type "NIH" in the search box and click on Google Search.

When the list of Web sites comes up, each will be followed by a short description of what it contains. The NIH site will come up first on the list or very near the top. Click on it, and you will get the home page. Then click on the first listing, "Health Information," then click on "P" for prostate. A list will come up including several topics for prostate matters. Click on "Prostate Diseases."

You will get a page headed "NIH Institutes and Center Resources." Below that you will find "National Institute of Diabetes, and Digestive and Kidney Diseases," with a list of subjects following. Some of these will deal with the prostate, because there is a medical connection with the urological system. You may click on a topic from this list. And *voila!* You have reached the information you wanted.

Another good place to start your research is WebMD.com. This Web site offers much information for free.

Get your information in stages

The total time you invest will depend on how fast you read and how many links you decide to investigate. Remember: Don't get bogged down in details. When you are satisfied that you have enough information to converse with your doctor, stop. You can always come back for more information after your next visit. While information is power, too much information can confuse you or scare you to death.

Internet research can help you fine-tune your conversations with your doctor, helping him help you. For instance, say you learned on the Internet that there is more than one type of mammogram. You can't ask your doctor which ones are available to you or ask him to compare them if you haven't learned this. Armed with his answer, you can better decide on one type that you both feel is better for you.

At this point, a word of warning: The amount of knowledge that you have acquired may make you giddy. Don't use it to impress your doctor. He may not appreciate it. But do use it to let him know you take your health seriously and are an informed patient. The Internet can provide you with information for better communication with your doctor on any subject. Learn to use it. It's not only helpful, it's fun.

I Can't Swallow That!
Prescriptions

6

Prescribing a pill for your problem is the fastest and easiest thing your doctor can do when you come to him with a complaint. Yet overmedication is one of the most serious problems in the health care of an aging population. The American Association of Retired Persons, whose membership is open to those over fifty, stated in a recent *AARP Bulletin* that more than four million older Americans take at least eight prescription drugs. It goes on to say that one in five Americans over sixty-five may be receiving improperly prescribed drugs. This does not include the over-the-counter supplements that patients may have added on their own.

The hype that bombards consumers through television and print advertising plants the idea that there is a pill for everything, sending patients to their doctors to ask for one (or more) of them.

In the Doctor's Office

There is not a pill for everything. A wise physician of another generation once looked at me when I arrived in his office with a miserable cold and said, "I know. You feel like hell, and there's not very much I can do about it." That was an honest answer. If your doctor gives you a "there's no pill" answer, don't force your way into that unnecessary overmedication trap. Ask him what will make you feel better, and follow his instructions.

Take a look at the Prescription Checklist in the Patient's Tool Kit at the back of this book. Use this list each time you meet with your doctor and get a prescription.

Side effects
Be sure you remind your doctor of any drug allergies.

"Kim" learned a lesson the hard way when she was

plagued with a stubborn sinus infection, which seemed to be affecting her ears and balance and upsetting her stomach with postnasal drainage. Since her ears were causing the most discomfort, she sought the advice of an ear specialist. He prescribed a course of antibiotics lasting thirty days. Almost immediately Kim developed other problems, many of which she assumed were symptoms of the still active infection. She ran a fever and had a headache. Her stomach was bloated and she burped excessively. These discomforts were followed by pain in her abdomen which spread around her back to the kidney area. She developed welts on her skin, and her feet swelled. She was miserable.

She went to see her primary-care physician, who prescribed a diuretic for the swelling feet, which she did not take.

When she returned to the doctor who was treating the sinus infection, he listened in stunned silence to her list of complaints. All of them, he explained, were possible side effects of the drug he had prescribed. They indicated an allergic reaction. "I was expecting to hear that you had to call 9-1-1," he admitted.

Kim was allergic to penicillin, having suffered a reaction more than forty years earlier. On the front of her folder was a red sticker indicating the allergy. The doctor missed it, and the drug he had prescribed was in the penicillin family. Although he apologized, that did nothing to alleviate the suffering she had endured.

There are "families" of drugs, for example the "statins" used to treat high cholesterol and ace-inhibitors, beta-blockers, and calcium-channel blockers used to treat high blood pressure. If the first drug your doctor prescribes for any ailment causes an allergic reaction, and he prescribes another, be sure to ask if it is in the same family and if it is likely that you will be allergic to it as well.

If you have any known allergies to specific substances, make it a point to ask your doctor every time he prescribes a new medication. Remember, he is seeing a host of patients. Your file gets thicker by the visit, and he does not carry this information in his head—you do.

Use your notepad

As he gives you the prescription, the doctor will probably say something like, "I want you to take two of these with food every morning for three days and then one with food in the evening for five days." Write this down. These instructions should be included in the information supplied by the pharmacy when you pick up the prescription, but they may not be. And you want to be sure that the instructions are the same. If they are not, call the doctor's office. There will be someone who can consult the chart to verify the orders. Improper use of medication is a major problem with aging patients.

Dosage is not something to be trusted to memory. You are not paying for the doctor's advice and laying out a bundle for the medicine so that you can inadvertently poison yourself.

If your doctor handwrites his prescriptions, look at what he has written. If you can't make out the letters in the name, the difference between *a* and *o* or between *r* and *n*, for example, ask for the spelling. Your pharmacist may not be able to make them out either. The doctor who generates his prescriptions by computer and turns them out on letter-size paper written in English makes it easier. If your doctor still uses Latin symbols, the chart on the next page may help.

The Food and Drug Administration (FDA) and the American Medical Association (AMA) have both urged more caution in writing prescriptions. Many drug names sound alike, and a mix-up can be serious. For example: Norvasc (amlodipine besylate) for high blood pressure sounds (and might look when handwritten) like Navane (thio-thixene) used to treat psychosis.

Levoxine (levothyroxine) for low thyroid looked and sounded so much like Lanoxin (digoxin) for heart failure, that the FDA requested that Levoxine's manufacturer change the name to Levoxyl.

If the prescription is for a drug regulated by the Federal Controlled Substances Act, the Drug Enforcement Administration requires the prescription contain your name and address, date, name of the drug, dosage, form (such as 5 milligram tablets), the amount the pharmacist may give you, directions for use, the number of refills, the doctor's name, address, DEA registration number, and his signature.

Your state may have additional regulations, such as requiring the label to say what the drug is to be used for. A number of states require this if the medication is given for a patient in a long-term care facility.

New medications

Just as you have an interest in what's new, so does your doctor. Ask if the medication he is prescribing has been recently developed. Remember the woman in the Versace suit with the Gucci attaché case who was sitting next to you in the waiting room? She was the representative of a major drug company, waiting for her chance to pitch the latest pharmaceuticals to your doctor. What is prescribed for you the next time you need medication may depend more on how good her pitch is rather than whether the new drug is more effective than the one you are taking. Of one thing be sure: It will cost more. And there is unlikely to be a generic equivalent.

A drug patent has a life span, and when it runs out other companies can make the drug. An available generic means that another company is making the equivalent medicine and charging less for it. If saving money is important, ask each time you get a refill if a generic has arrived on the market. If one has, ask your doctor if he feels it is all right to switch.

If your doctor prescribes a new medicine to replace the one you are taking, your first question should be to yourself, "Is the one I am taking working?" And to him, "How will this drug be better and why?" If the new drug costs more, discuss the cost/benefit ratio with the doctor.

Doctors are not any more immune to advertising hype and sales pitches than consumers. There is also the allure of the new. If the doctor is convinced that a new drug is better than the one you are taking, he may prescribe it. In this case, it is up to you to watch closely to see if it really is better for you.

Ask your doctor if he has a sample of the medication. Drug companies routinely supply samples to doctors. Some doctors offer them to patients. Some don't. A sample may help you determine within a day or two if the medicine does not agree with you. If you are really ill, it will allow you to go to the pharmacy after you start feeling better.

When your doctor suggests a medicine, ask him whether he is prescribing the maximum dosage, the minimum, or something in between. Treatment theories differ. Some doctors will prescribe the maximum with the intention of cutting the dosage if it produces symptoms that the patient cannot tolerate. Some prescribe the minimum and increase the dosage if it does not produce the desired results. You should know which yours prefers.

You may never know what influences your doctor to prescribe one medicine over another, but there is no reason (except that pesky time limit)

Latin prescription terms

Abbreviation	Latin	Meaning
a.c.	ante cibum	before meals
b.i.d	bis in die	twice a day
gtt	guttae	drops
h.s.	hora somni	at bedtime
od	oculus dexter	right eye
os	oculus sinister	left eye
po	per os	by mouth
p.c.	post cibum	after meals
prn	pro re nata	as needed
q3h	quaque 3 hora	every three hours
qd	quaque die	every day
qid	quater in die	4 times a day
tid	ter in die	3 times a day

you can't ask him. Perhaps he has a history of prescribing it and is comfortable with the results. Or he may have read an article in a medical journal detailing the results of clinical trials. Such articles became more suspect after the year 2000, when *The New England Journal of Medicine* was revealed to have violated its own policy of not allowing authors who have financial ties to a drug manufacturer to write reviews and expert opinions.

Asking for a Prescription by Phone

"If you are sick, you should make an appointment to be seen," a doctor explained. "When the patient calls and says, 'I know I have ailment X, and I need the doctor to call in a prescription for medication Y for me,' he makes the doctor responsible for the diagnosis and the treatment without ever having seen the patient."

There was once a time when you could call your primary-care physician and ask for a prescription if you were ill. Malpractice suits have ended this. Unless you are asking for a refill, the doctor is unlikely to prescribe medication without seeing you. If it has been a long time since he saw you, he may refuse anyway.

The Pharmacy

There is a second line of defense and that is the pharmacist who fills your prescription. His years of education and professional practice have been devoted solely to drugs. He is the expert. Your doctor may actually suggest you check with your pharmacist if you have additional questions. Even if your doctor was thorough in explaining about your medication, it is a good idea to go through it again with your pharmacist.

$$R_x$$

What does the R_x on the prescription pad mean? One theory is that it is an abbreviation of the Latin word *recipe*, which means "take." A more romantic theory is that it represents the astrological sign of Jupiter, which was placed on ancient prescriptions to invoke the blessing of that powerful god to help the medicine make the patient well.

You don't have to buy a whole prescription at once. The pharmacy will sell you any portion you want and keep the information on file so that you can get the rest of it at any time. Often a week's supply is sufficient to test a new medication for adverse reactions. That way, if you have a reaction, you won't end up discarding a full bottle of expensive pills.

Another reason you may want to get less than a full prescription is to spread the cost of a prescription into the next month. Just be sure buying your prescriptions piecemeal doesn't create havoc with your insurance company.

Refills

What about refills? Doctors have put prescription renewals on a time schedule, too. More and more doctors don't want to take the time to rewrite a prescription when you run out. As a doctor interviewed about prescriptions explained, "If you call needing a refill of your prescription because you are completely out, it may be difficult to get that medication for you in a timely manner."

Know if your doctor has a schedule for writing refill prescriptions. He may post a sign reminding you that refill prescriptions will be written only on a certain day of the week or when you come in for an appointment. If you take medication for an ongoing condition, your physician may write a prescription at the time of your annual physical. It saves your time and his to ask for it then. Part of your preparation for any appointment should be to check your supply of medicines so you can ask for renewals if you need them.

The number of refills your doctor considers appropriate will be noted on the prescription and on the label the pharmacist puts on the bottle. Watch that number. You don't want to run out on a weekend,when you cannot simply go to the pharmacy for a refill.

Prescription Problems and Possible Solutions

Problem	Possible Solutions
Impaired vision	• Ask pharmacist to use large print on label. • Use a magnifying glass to check labels before taking medications.
Impaired hearing	• Let others know if you did not hear the instructions. • Ask doctor/pharmacist to write instructions. • Ask someone to go with you to the doctor.
Complex dosage schedule	• Write down your schedule clearly and use color to differentiate times of day. Use daily/weekly medication dispensers. Coordinate the time to take medication with specific activities (e.g., meal time, time of favorite television program, when mail arrives, etc.).

Forgetfulness	• Use memory aids and daily or weekly medication dispensers.
	• Place notes to yourself where you will see them.
Limited mobility	• Use a pharmacy that will deliver prescriptions (cost may be higher).
Limited use of hands	• Ask pharmacist for easy-to-open bottle caps.
Multiple medications	• Have doctor evaluate medication regimen regularly.
	• Use a pharmacy that keeps a patient profile for customers.
Multiple doctors	• Make sure each doctor knows all medications you are taking.
	• Purchase all prescriptions at only one pharmacy.
Cost of medications	• Call local pharmacies and compare prices.
	• Ask doctor or pharmacist whether a generic drug will be as effective and less costly.
	• Ask doctor or pharmacist if you qualify for a patient assistance program through a drug company.

Filling Prescriptions in other Countries

With the exploding cost of prescription drugs, controversy rages about where to buy medicine. At this writing, Canadian pharmacies offer U.S. citizens lower prices and have become major players in the mail order business. This practice borders on the illegal in the U.S. and may not remain an option. If you are a U.S. citizen and happen to live within driving distance of the Canadian border, you can buy your drugs in Canada in person. You might hop on a bus with a group of friends and party your way to and from with part of the money you save.

The same applies to Mexico. Mail order business from Mexico into the United States does not flourish, but residents of the U.S. who live within driving distance of that border seek the savings that are available at the Mexican pharmacies. Some who winter in the border areas manage to collect a year's supply during their winter vacations. There are border towns whose existence depends on parking lots full of motor coaches belonging to snowbirds who stock up on medications and other goodies while they are in the neighborhood.

Although in some Mexican border towns you do not need a prescription to purchase some drugs—the pharmacy will want to see one for barbiturates and narcotics—it is a good idea to have all prescriptions in hand. Currently, Customs at the Mexican border allows you to bring a three-month supply of any given drug into the U.S. Try to bring more and you may have to turn around and take it back.

If you are planning to use one of these sources for your medicine, will you be safe? You decide. Many times these medicines are manufactured in the United States. Others are manufactured in Europe, in countries that have illustrious records of good medicinal quality. A sensible question that I heard a patient ask during a discussion about the safety of foreign-bought drugs was, "Do you mean to tell me that U.S. drug manufacturers are selling substandard medicines to our good friends in Canada?"

Still, controls are stringent in the United States, and they may be lacking in other nations.

Medicare

Medicare has made a prescription drug program available to any Medicare beneficiary. On its Web site, medicare.gov, you will find a complete description of the program and the tools for figuring out how much the program will cost you. Before you start, know how much you are paying for drugs per year or how much help you receive if you have a prescription drug program already in place through your pension or insurance plan. The December 2005 issue of the *AARP Bulletin* contains an article outlining how to use the site. You can access the AARP eight-page question-and-answer guide at aarp.org/bulletin/medicarerx. That Web site links to a worksheet designed to help you make a choice.

The Scary, Expensive, Amazing, Wonderful World of Tests

"The XYZ test will tell us if you need a PDQ test. Just take this to the lab on Dooley Street."

You may encounter similar statements in your doctor's office, and when you do, you need to be ready with your questions—what, why, and how much.

As the foremost advocate for your health care, you want to be sure that the tests your doctor orders are necessary and potentially beneficial.

If you ask your questions without challenging your doctor's motives or his authority, he should not be put off. You are entitled to know the ramifications of what your doctor is suggesting.

This is another time to pull out your notebook. Start by writing down the name of the test. If you are unsure of the spelling, ask. Be sure to record the answers to each of your other questions too.

Deal with the *why* first. Ask what your doctor has uncovered in his examination that he needs to verify by further testing. He should be able to give you a clear answer. If he has found a lump or a mass that needs further investigation, or if you have a symptom that is commonly tied to a specific ailment, he should describe the possibilities. Some doctors skip this, claiming that they do not want to worry a patient unnecessarily. Not knowing is one major cause of worry. Avoiding the truth doesn't help. To participate in your own health-care decisions you need complete information. Questions to Ask If Your Doctor Wants to Order Tests in the Patient's Tool Kit at the back of this book will help.

Tests don't cure anything. They are used as an aid in diagnosis. Some doctors are test happy. Ordering another test gets you out of the office faster and puts some of the burden on another health-care professional or at least postpones discussion until another day. It saves the physician's time, but not yours. If your doctor is the aggressive type, he may be inclined to order more tests in his eagerness to get to the bottom of your problem or to satisfy his curiosity. If it seems that the doctor is ordering an excessive number of tests, ask more questions. He may be trying to cover all possible eventualities to avoid being accused of missing something.

Your first question should be, "What is this test going to tell us?" It could be used to confirm a diagnosis that the doctor already suspects based on what he has observed. It could be used to cross-check the results of a previous test. If you are already being treated, it could be used to indicate the need for a change in treatment or medication.

There are a number of simple tests that doctors have been using for years. You may have had some of them as part of a routine physical examination: chest x-rays, electrocardiogram, urinalysis, and blood screening.

New, noninvasive tests are being developed every day. Even if you had a test in the past, procedures and instruments may have been modified and improved in the interim.

New Equipment

Have you ever bought a new gadget? You couldn't wait to get it out of box and find out how it worked, could you? The world of tests can affect doctors the same way.

Many tests are performed by machines that cost millions of dollars. They are generally owned by private imaging companies or by hospitals, and sometimes by a consortium of doctors working in cooperation with a hospital. These entities fully expect to pay for the machines and make a profit.

As these new tests become available, your doctor will want to use them to better care for you. You will need to ask the questions that will assure that it is the best job. Be sure that tried and true tests are not passed up for the opportunity to deliver you into the hands of new space-age machinery.

Does your doctor know the cost of this test and whether your health insurance will pay for it? Some new tests cost several thousand dollars each. Is the test experimental? Insurance companies sometimes back away from experimental procedures. You will want to check with your insurance company to be sure the test is covered. You'll also want to know what portion of the cost you'll be expected to pay.

Talking to your doctor about a sophisticated test is often difficult within the time limit of a regular office appointment. There's the danger you may not learn enough about it. Don't agree to a test until you are comfortable with the amount of information you have.

Twenty-four Common Tests Your Doctor May Suggest

Three terms that appear in the descriptions of many tests should be explained:

- *Fluoroscopy* is a technique for taking "live" x-rays. An x-ray beam is transmitted through the patient and strikes a fluorescent plate that is connected to an image intensifier, which is connected to a television camera. The radiologist can view the images live on a monitor.
- *Contrast material* or *contrast dye* is a substance or dye used to make images appear more visible on x-rays, and may be used with other procedures. Iodine and barium are two that are often used.
- A *transducer* is a device used to change energy from one system to another, from electrical impulse to sound, for example.

   ANGIOGRAM—This x-ray test, using fluoroscopy, takes pictures of the blood flow in an artery or a vein. A catheter (a thin, flexible tube) is placed in an artery in the groin or above the elbow and guided to the spot to be studied. A dye containing iodine is injected into the blood vessel to make it show more clearly in the x-ray. This test, with some degrees of modification, can be used for areas of the heart, lung, or brain.

   ARTERIAL BLOOD GASES (ABG)—This test measures the levels of oxygen and carbon dioxide in your blood to determine how well your lungs move oxygen into your blood and remove carbon dioxide. Blood is drawn from an artery usually in the wrist where oxygen and carbon dioxide levels can be measured before they are changed by entering body tissues. Other gases in the blood are measured as well, but changes in oxygen and carbon dioxide can indicate changes in the function of the heart, circulation, lungs, and kidneys.

BARIUM ENEMA—The colon is filled with liquid containing barium and an x-ray examination of the large intestine follows. Barium makes the x-ray images clearer.

BARIUM SWALLOW—Upper gastrointestinal series (UGI)—you will swallow the barium with water, often with gas-producing crystals. The doctor will use fluoroscopy connected to a video monitor to track the barium through your esophagus, stomach, and the first part of the small intestine. A small bowel follow-through may be done immediately after to examine the entire length of the small intestine.

BIOPSY—This is the surgical removal of sample tissue from the body for examination for diagnostic purposes. Since tissue is examined microscopically, samples can be small.

BLOOD GLUCOSE TEST—Blood is drawn and measured for the amount of glucose (a type of sugar) in your blood. Most common is the fasting blood sugar test done after you have fasted for at least eight hours. It is often the first test given if diabetes is suspected.

COMPLETE BLOOD COUNT—Your blood reveals many things about your condition. Blood is drawn and examined to determine the number of red blood cells, white blood cells, and platelets. This information helps your doctor determine what is causing bruising or weakness. It also aids in diagnosing anemia, infection and other problems. An expanded *blood screen* also tests for kidney and liver function, cholesterol, and triglycerides.

BONE MINERAL DENSITY (BMD)—These tests measure the loss of minerals, such as calcium, from your bones. This loss can lead to osteoporosis, which is more common in women over sixty-five, but men can suffer from it too. There are several methods to measure bone loss, but dual-energy x-ray absorptionmetry (DEXA) can measure bone loss as little as 2 percent a year. It uses low doses of radiation from two different x-ray beams to measure the bone density in your hips and spine. It is fast and painless.

BONE SCAN—This is a nuclear scanning test, where a radioactive tracer is injected into a vein in the arm. It takes about three hours for this to move through your body. You will then be positioned under a large scanning camera, which will take pictures from all angles. The camera produces no radiation. A bone scan can detect areas of bone growth or breakdown and cancer that has metastasized to the bone. It offers earlier detection than a regular x-ray.

COMPUTED TOMOGRAPHY (CT or CAT SCAN)—The patient lies on a table attached to a machine that is like a giant doughnut. The table moves through the doughnut hole as the machine sends a series of x-rays through the body. Each pulse takes a picture of a thin slice of the organ or area of the body and saves them on a computer for examination. A CT scan can be used to examine many parts of the body. It can be used with iodine dye or barium swallow as a contrast material.

MAGNETIC RESONANCE IMAGING (MRI)—For this test you will lie on a table that slides into a large tube-like machine until the part of your body being imaged is inside the machine. The machine uses a powerful magnetic field and radio waves to make pictures of organs and tissues. Contrast material may be used to get better pictures. An MRI can often give better information than an x-ray, CT scan, or ultrasound. The machine is very noisy.

ULTRASOUND (DOPPLER ULTRASOUND)—This test uses sound waves to evaluate the blood vessels or organs that are being studied. The person administering the test will use a hand-held transducer that is passed lightly over the skin above the site. It uses reflected sound waves that are processed by a computer into images which can be saved for future examination. The test is painless.

PULMONARY FUNCTION TESTS (PFT)—There are a number of these tests all designed to find out how well your lungs work. Usually, the first test done is *spirometry*. This measures how much air you move in and out of your lungs and how quickly. You will breathe into a mouthpiece attached to a spirometer, which collects the information and prints it out on a chart for your doctor to examine. Additional specialized tests may be ordered also.

PROSTATE-SPECIFIC ANTIGEN (PSA)—This blood test for men only measures the amount of prostate-specific antigen in the blood. High levels of PSA may indicate problems with the prostate gland that are determined through additional tests.

MAMMOGRAM—A mammogram is an x-ray of the breasts. It is used as a diagnostic tool for early detection of breast cancer. It can also detect other abnormalities in the breast—cysts or benign lumps. Digital mammograms are a different imaging technique. Each has advantages.

BREAST CANCER BRCA GENE TEST—A BRCA gene test is a blood test for women with a strong family history of breast cancer, or in some cases women who have already had breast cancer. It provides a risk analysis for women who have the BRCA1 or the BRCA2 gene.

ELECTROENCEPHALOGRAM (EEG)—An EEG measures and records the electrical activity in the brain through electrodes attached to your head and connected to a computer. Changes such as seizures can be detected when they show up in the normal pattern of brain activity.

COLONOSCOPY—This test enables your doctor to examine the interior of your rectum and large intestine. He uses a thin, flexible tube, a colonoscope, to help detect polyps, bleeding ulcers, and tumors. The patient is given liquid or pills, or a combination to clean out the colon before the examination. A light anesthetic is given.

PAP TEST—This test for women only is used for early detection of cervical cancer. The doctor collects a small cell sample from the surface of the cervix and sends it to a lab to be examined for abnormalities, cancer cells, or changes that could lead to cancer. PAP tests should be scheduled regularly—ask your doctor.

COLPOSCOPY AND CERVICAL BIOPSY—If PAP test results are abnormal, the doctor may use a colposcope to get a magnified view of the vagina and cervix. It can be used with a camera for a permanent record. A small sample of tissue is taken for microscopic examination.

Cardiac tests

There are many heart tests. The following are often used:

ELECTROCARDIOGRAM (EKG)—This test measures the electrical impulses that control the rhythm of the patient's heartbeat. Small metal disks called electrodes are attached to the skin and connected to a machine that converts the activity of the heart into lines traced on paper. The machine can translate these tracings, which the doctor then reviews to detect heart problems.

ECHOCARDIOGRAM—This is a type of ultrasound test using high pitched sound waves to produce an image of the heart. Again, a transducer is used and the sound waves are reflected from the heart and converted to pictures on a video monitor. This test checks the heart wall and the heart valves, whether the heart is contracting normally and whether there is a blood clot or damage to the heart.

STRESS TEST (exercise electrocardiogram, treadmill test)—A resting electrocardiogram is done before a stress test to be sure that there are no problems that would make the stress test unsafe. The patient walks on a treadmill or rides a stationary bicycle to place the heart under stress. This test detects coronary artery disease, which results in poor blood flow to the heart.

CARDIAC PERFUSION SCAN—A radioactive tracer is injected into a vein in the patient's arm. A gamma camera shows the tracer moving through the heart. If there is poor blood flow to areas of the heart, the tracer will not be absorbed, indicating blocked blood vessels or a previous heart attack. The procedure may involve both resting images and stress images. If patient cannot walk on a treadmill, the heart is stressed with medication.

Your biggest question is probably What are they going to do to me? Is any part of it invasive? Will they inject me with dye or any other substance to facilitate the test? Will anesthetic be necessary or anything that might preclude going to the test alone or impair my ability to drive? Will I have to be hospitalized for the procedure?

Be Attentive to Details

Risk

Ask if there is an element of risk. Most tests are safe, but some include a small risk factor. You may be asked to sign a waiver before the test promising not to sue if something goes awry. Get your doctor to spell out what, if any, the risks are. Ask what may happen if you decide not to have the test. This will help you weigh the risks against the benefits.

Find out where the test will be given. In a major urban area, the facility may be close by. Some testing devices are so new and so expensive that if you live in a small city or a rural area, you may have to travel a great distance to have the test done. Be sure to get the telephone number of the hospital or imaging center so you can call ahead verify the appointment.

How long will the actual test take? Some tests include breaks—stress tests, for example. Some tests take more than one day. If the test will require that you be given an anesthetic, find out how long it will last. If you need to rearrange your schedule or ask a friend or relative to be with you, you will need time to plan. It can strain a friendship if you assure the person waiting that you will be finished in an hour, only to awake two hours later still on the gurney in recovery.

Ask when the test results will be available and how you will get them. The doctor may want you to make an appointment to receive the results in person, or he may have someone in his office telephone you.

Don't rush

Don't be stampeded, either by your doctor or by your own feelings. Most tests can be safely postponed for a day or two. This will give you time to read up on the procedure. Ask your doctor if he has any printed material he can give you, and check your library or bookstore. Do some Internet research. You may wish to talk to someone who has had this test, but don't rely too heavily on their opinions unless they are medical professionals.

Information on many tests is available from the National Institutes of Health Web site, nih.gov. An Internet site called How Stuff Works, howstuffworks.com, has a great description of how an MRI machine works.

Informed decisions

As you know, doctors differ. Some have a more conservative wait-and-see approach to tests. This may be your preference too. If it is, it is still important for you to learn what tests are available, what information they may provide, what risks, if any, are associated with a particular test, and what costs come into play. Only then can you make an informed decision.

Using a specialist

Some tests are best done under a specialist's supervision. When a heart test requires a physician to be present, the physician should be a cardiologist. Neurological tests should be supervised by a neurologist. The reason is that a specialist may get additional information by observing the patient.

Avoiding repeat tests

No one wants to undergo a test only to have to have it repeated. If your doctor orders a test that is to be reviewed by another doctor, perhaps a specialist, contact the specialist to see how he wants the test conducted. And remember, often it is best if the specialist supervises the test.

Preparing for your test

If the appointment is made through your physician's office, they will notify you of the time and location of the test. If special instructions or advance procedures such as fasting are necessary, the doctor's staff should inform you accordingly. The testing agency may call you to verify that you understood the instructions and to answer any last-minute questions you may have. Write everything down. Don't trust your memory. You could lose precious time or skew the results if you omit any test preliminaries.

When you arrive at the lab for your test, ask the technicians what they are going to do. These professionals are proud of what they do and are often more than willing to explain procedures to you. They can tell you very quickly while they are dialing in last-minute settings on the machine or putting a clean sheet on the examining table. They can help eliminate any lingering apprehension over the test.

Many tests must be interpreted by a specialist. The specialist will then relay the results to your physician. Some tests are read by more than one person. For instance many facilities that give mammograms have at least two radiologists read them to reduce the possibility of errors. In any event, technicians will usually leave the evaluation of the test to others and decline to give you much information.

Getting the results

Test results tend to get lost in the shuffle, so patients often wait longer than necessary to learn the results. Five to seven business days is usually long enough. If you haven't heard from the doctor in a reasonable length of time, don't assume anything, either good or bad. Call and find out.

As always, take notes. Make sure you understand the results of a test. Is a "positive" result good and a "negative" result bad, or vice versa? If you are high on a scale, is that reason to celebrate or reason to take drastic action?

Elective testing

When every media-mention of health-care trumpets the benefits of early detection and everyone around you seems to be having tests for one symptom or another, you may become concerned and think you need a test. As you know, your physician is the best person to consult on the need for testing. Most will be reluctant to order tests that they feel are purely elective.

But there has been, in recent years, a growing market of full-body CT scans performed by independent companies. These tests are touted in advertisements as early detection devices that provide you with the peace of mind that one problem or another is not going undetected.

These scans are somewhat expensive. Without a doctor's order, Medicare and many health plans will not cover them. They are also controversial. Doctors are divided in their opinions of full-body scans as a diagnostic tool. The scan sends radiation through the body and, properly read by a specialist, can detect tumors, cysts, and aneurysms measuring into the hundredths of an inch. However, they also show "spots" that may be scars from healed infections and other harmless abnormalities, causing unwarranted alarm.

A full-body scan might alert you to a problem, but you will be subjecting your body to considerably more radiation than is received from an x-ray, and you may be spending money unnecessarily. These are factors that need to be weighed against whatever comfort you feel you might get from a full-body scan.

A list of questions to ask if your doctor wants to schedule tests for you is in the Patient's Tool Kit at the back of this book. Either photocopy the questions or take the book along to your appointment with the page marked.

8

It Sometimes Comes to this: "You need surgery."

The first step toward having surgery is to have ruled out the alternatives to having surgery.

Some alternatives may be more onerous than the surgery itself. These include serious side effects that accompany some medications and the prospect of living the rest of your life with pain. But many times, alternatives exist that will allow you to avoid going under the knife.

Many of today's less invasive surgeries require little or no recovery time. Yet no surgery is entirely without risk. Be sure you and your doctor rule out any viable alternatives before agreeing to surgery.

Naturally some anxiety is connected to the decision to have surgery. This can be lessened by learning about the procedure and being prepared. Again, do your research, take a list of written questions to your doctor, and take notes as he answers them.

Selecting a surgeon is of utmost importance. One way is to get a recommendation from your primary-care physician. Whom does he recommend to perform the surgery and why? Would he go to this surgeon if he were having the same surgery? Has he referred a number of patients to the surgeon with good results? Can he arrange for you to talk with a patient who has had the same procedure?

Is the doctor suggesting a general surgeon or a subspecialist, such as a cardiac surgeon? It is unlikely that you will find a surgeon who performs only appendectomies, but a doctor who focuses on one type of surgery is usually the best choice. Many operations require a high degree of expertise, and you want a surgeon with a long and successful record of doing the particular operation you'll be undergoing.

If you choose not to ask for a referral from your current doctor, use the strategies for finding a doctor discussed in Chapter 1.

As with any doctor, if you wish to investigate a surgeon, the Internet can help. You can find licensing information for doctors in your state, sometimes including the number of legal or medical board actions that may be pending against a particular doctor. Usually the details of the actions will not be listed. Some sites include the doctor's educational background. If you are concerned about any of what you find, discuss your concerns with your primary-care physician or some other knowledgeable person. See Web Sites of Interest at the back of this book.

The selection of a surgeon is a highly personal one. You are conceivably placing your life in this person's hands. Surgery is worrisome enough by itself. You should have no concerns about the skill or dedication of your surgeon. Don't dwell on personality flaws. As Dr. Wesley Johnson, a busy Arizona surgeon who specializes in advanced spine and orthopedic surgery, points out, "The best doctor is not always the sweetest one with the flashiest smile."

Enter the Surgeon

"A surgeon is more defined in his role and more narrow in his focus than your primary-care physician," says Dr. Johnson. "A surgeon is probably not interested in your life story. A good thing to do is to write down your history and bring it with you prior to surgery. Include major health problems and diagnoses. One typed page is best. Random thoughts and subjective conversation are rarely productive."

The surgeon can read your one-page written history—see How to Create a One Page Medical History in the Patient's Tool Kit at the back of the book for what to include—faster than you can tell him, and if he has any questions, he will know what to ask. "In training we are taught to listen to the patients and to lead them into productive conversation," Johnson explains. "If your surgeon does not appear to be listening to you, perhaps he is trying to lead you into giving him more precise information."

In addition to the *dos* of bringing your one-page history and your list of questions to the appointment, Dr. Johnson offers this list of *don'ts*:

- Don't walk in and ask for a pain medication. You may appear to be looking for drugs.

- Don't complain about another doctor—"He doesn't know what he's talking about." "He's poorly trained." "He doesn't listen."

The American Board of Medical Specialties recognizes the following twenty-four fields of medical specialties:

- Allergy and immunology
- Anesthesiology
- Colon and rectal surgery
- Dermatology
- Emergency medicine
- Family medicine
- Internal medicine
- Medical genetics
- Neurological surgery
- Nuclear medicine
- Obstetrics and gynecology
- Ophthalmology
- Orthopaedic surgery
- Otolaryngology
- Pathology
- Pediatrics
- Physical medicine and rehabilitation
- Plastic surgery
- Preventive medicine
- Psychiatry and neurology
- Radiology
- Surgery
- Thoracic surgery
- Urology

- Never mention an attorney. This raises a flag that you are thinking of potential wrongdoing or malpractice.

- Don't display hostility, aggressiveness, or anger or take a hostile family member with you. A family member has every bit as much influence on the doctor as the patient.

- Don't ask for a guarantee. Some patients demand a guarantee, suggesting unrealistic expectations.

The patient/surgeon relationship

Dr. Johnson likens the relationship between a patient and a surgeon to a marriage, explaining that anesthesia, surgery, and aftercare are meaningful involvements that create a spiritual bond, like a marriage. Certainly, most actions in the "don'ts" list above would stress a marriage.

Examine your expectations as far as this surgery is concerned. "Most of the falling out between a surgeon and a patient is caused by over-expectations," Johnson says. Your expectations should guide the questions you ask. Johnson offers the following:

- Ask if this will be inpatient or outpatient surgery. Find out how long the hospital stay will be for inpatient surgery. Ask if outpatient surgery means you'll have to stay all day.

- If you are in poor general health, ask, "What are my chances of surviving this surgery?"

- Ask what the biggest risks of complications are and what the most common complications are.

- Ask how long it might be before you will feel reasonably good and how long before you will be completely healed. (These are two different questions and will probably get two different answers.)

Many surgeries that once required days in the hospital don't even require one night's stay. Some are done in the doctor's office. If you will need to go to a hospital and you prefer a certain hospital, ask if the surgery can be done there. Your surgeon may have privileges at more than one hospital and may be happy to accommodate your wishes.

Ask for details of the operation. "A part of what doctors learn in their training is how to make medical terms understandable in lay language," Dr. Johnson says. "If you don't understand, you can always ask your surgeon to use an analogy."

How much detail do you want to hear? Dr. Johnson believes that detail confuses and frightens some patients. If you are fascinated by detail, ask your doctor to explain in detail. On the other hand, if you think you'll feel queasy or be disturbed by a detailed explanation, go for the simple one. The full color posters, flip carts, and plaster models in many surgeons' offices are useful tools for the doctor to use in describing the problem and the procedure. You can use them to help illustrate your questions too.

With major surgeries, you may need blood transfusions. If this is the case, ask if you should stockpile your own blood to be used.

Anesthetics

Another valid question concerns the anesthetic your surgeon will use. If you have had previous surgeries, you may know what worked best for you. If you were given something that put you down for two days, discuss this with him. If you had a wicked sore throat following a surgery it might have been caused by a tube inserted in your throat. Mention this to your surgeon or the anesthesiologist and ask that steps be taken so it doesn't happen again. If you have knowledge of the anesthesiologists in your area and have a preference, ask if you can make the choice.

Plan Ahead

Have a recovery plan. Discuss your recovery at your pre-op appointment. Think about your day-to-day activities in connection with your recovery. Prepare a list of written questions for this appointment. You will want to know if there are restrictions on actions you make, such as bending over, reaching up, picking up a toddler, running the vacuum cleaner, or lifting anything heavier than a coffee cup. It can be an unpleasant surprise to find out that the procedure has left you unable to put on your socks or comb your hair.

Questions you'll want to ask may include: How much help from others will I need? When will I be able to drive my car, go back to work, or get back to my exercise routine?

If you are an ardent hobbyist, you may have an extra set of questions centered around the special demands your hobby makes on your body. When will you be able to use your drill press, sew a quilt, climb a mountain, paddle a kayak, or kneel down to garden? Tailor your questions to the specific requirements of your lifestyle.

Find out if your surgery will require post-operation therapy. If so, you will want to ask when it will begin, what it will include, how long it is likely to last, and where it will be conducted. While at the doctor's office, ask for a preprinted sheet of post-op instructions. Work these instructions and the answers to your questions into your recovery plan.

Informed consent

You will be given a number of documents by your surgeon, some to sign and some to read. Important among them will be an informed consent or surgical disclosure form. You should take ample time to read it, and be sure you understand it. Often it is handed to you at the close of your pre-op appointment when you are already on information overload. The tendency at this point is to skim it and sign it, thinking you have probably covered everything in it already. Since you know it is coming, ask for it when you first arrive in the office, explaining that you would like to use your time waiting to be sure you understand it.

The form may include a description of the proposed surgery and certain disclosures. By signing it, you may be agreeing to one or more of the following:

- That you have discussed and understand the possible risks and complications for the proposed surgery.

- That alternative treatments have been explained to you.

- That your surgeon may use assistants as he deems appropriate.

- That you authorize the doctor and his assistants to provide such additional procedures as they deem necessary.

- That blood transfusions are authorized and used at the discretion of the doctor or the staff.

- The method of disposal of any tissues removed during the surgery.

Waivers of certain rights may be included. It is important that you be given time to read this form and that you understand it. Ask questions. If you feel rushed, ask to take it with you, specifying when you'll return with it.

Discuss any objections you have to signing the document with your doctor or the doctor's staff.

Pain

Pain is a major concern of surgical patients. Discuss pain control with your surgeon before you go to the hospital. Ask to be given a prescription for pain medication at your pre-op appointment so that you can have it on hand when you get home from the hospital. Otherwise you may be scrambling to have someone pick up the medicine for you, enduring a delay before you get it. Also be sure to make arrangements for refills if they will be needed.

The hospital

There are some things you can do ahead of time that will help reduce the stress of a hospital visit.

You can often check the rating and mortality rate of a hospital by contacting your state's medical quality assurance board by phone or via the Internet. You can visit the hospital if you are not familiar with it. Just seeing the inside of the building may make you feel more comfortable. You can usually walk the halls at will, so long as you stay out of areas marked "Employees Only." Or you can almost always find a hospital auxiliary volunteer to take you on a tour.

On the day of your surgery you will probably be asked to arrive very early. If you don't function until you have had your first cup of coffee, too bad. You won't have been allowed to eat or drink anything since at least midnight.

There are a few things you can do to make the morning of your surgery go more smoothly. Call the hospital admitting office and tell them what day you are scheduled for surgery. Ask if they would be willing to take all the admitting information before the day of your surgery.

Mark Yourself with an Eyebrow Pencil

If the surgeon is scheduled to remove something you have two of—a breast, a leg, a kidney—take an eyebrow pencil with you to the hospital and mark the one that is to remain with "Save this one" and the other with "Take this one." Don't use an "X." It might suggest a target. Sometimes the pre-op nurse will ask you to mark the site of a lump or a pain, but if she doesn't, you mark it.

In some cases you may need to report to the hospital the day before for a blood test, and you can do the paperwork at the same time.

Take along your medical history. The hospital is going to ask you for it. They will also want to know if you have a living will and/or a health-care power of attorney. If you do, take along copies for their files.

One of the documents you are asked to sign is the hospital privacy policy, designed to protect your medical information from prying eyes—behemoth data-gathering services. Be sure to list on the form friends or family members whom you wish to have access to your information. Once you have signed this form for a hospital, it should be in the system and find its way to the hospital records department. This would enable any of the persons you authorized to get a copy of the records of any procedures the hospital has performed for you.

It doesn't always work that way. Often you will sign a privacy statement for each procedure separately. This naturally complicates matters. If you need a hospital record and are unable to go for it yourself, the person you send should be prepared to track down the signed release form. Always ask for copies of any forms you sign. This practice may prove invaluable more than a few times.

While you are filling out the forms, ask the hospital for a copy of the Patients' Bill of Rights. Developed by the American Hospital Association in 1971, the Patients' Bill of Rights is distributed by many hospitals. As the name implies, it lists the things you have a right to expect as a patient. Some hospitals publish this along with a list of patients' responsibilities.

With the paperwork done, you can report directly to the surgery area on the morning of the operation.

It is a good idea to leave all valuables at home. You won't need a purse or wallet, but don't forget your identification and insurance cards. Wear comfortable clothes and shoes.

The Day of the Surgery

Admission into a hospital is somewhat degrading, depersonalizing, and it can be frightening. You will be given a bracelet that seemingly reduces your identity to a number. You will be asked to remove your clothes and given one of those little cover-ups that never quite do the job. Someone will show up with a clipboard and ask again all the questions that you answered yesterday. Additional documents will be produced for you to sign. A staff member will probably draw blood. Next, someone will put an intravenous needle in your arm. You may be given a shot to relax you. (This is a good thing.) Just try to stay calm and go with the flow.

In time you'll find yourself lying atop a gurney being pushed by someone in scrubs. Your chauffeur will fly down hallways, race in and out of elevators, and whip around corners, while you wonder why they don't put artwork on the ceiling. You will know you have reached the operating room when the temperature drops fifteen degrees.

There will likely be a gang of masked people in the operating room, calmly talking about what they did last weekend or gossiping over some hospital intrigue. About now you will see the anesthesiologist, as he bends over and asks you to count backward from 100, or to pick out your dream, or maybe to just say "good night."

You will miss the ensuing procedures and may or may not remember anything about the recovery room. Eventually you will wake up in your room, probably a bit groggy, but happy to have the surgery behind you.

Dr. Johnson adds a word to the wise about your hospital stay: "It is the nurse who will take care of you, and patients develop important relationships with their nurse. There may not always be a good match of personalities. If for some reason you have a nurse that you cannot get along with, there is almost always a head nurse or floor supervisor. Ask for her and explain the problem. She can assign another nurse."

In some hospitals you may be assigned a case manager. Find out who that person is. A good many of your questions can be answered by her. Good communication is the key to making your hospital visit the best possible experience.

You will see your surgeon when he makes hospital rounds, but you may be sleeping or partially sedated when he comes in. If you have a question you want answered before you leave the hospital, ask the nurse what time he usually makes his rounds and ask your spouse or a friend to be there with you at that time. With two of you to listen and one of you to write down information, you can be sure of better results from the meeting.

9

Getting a Second Opinion

When your doctor has presented you with a bleak diagnosis, is suggesting that you undergo a significant surgical procedure, or is advocating that you begin a long-term course of medication, you may wish to obtain a second opinion. You have this right and, if there is the slightest bit of doubt, you owe it to yourself to do so. You also owe it to your family members who want to see you get the best care available. And, besides, your insurance company may require it before committing to an expensive bill.

Telling the doctor you want to get a second opinion might feel awkward to you, but he will have been presented with this situation before, and most physicians are highly understanding. Your doctor may even beat you to the punch and suggest it himself. It is likely he has been on the other end and has been consulted for second opinions. It is also likely that he would do the same thing if he or one of his family members were in your shoes.

If your doctor gives you a bad time or tries to talk you out of seeking a second opinion, you may want to take a hard look at your relationship with him.

If your doctor says, "I wouldn't wait," ask him how much time he feels *is* safe. Unless he's about to hustle you off to the hospital in an ambulance, you are likely to have a few days to get another consultation. If he says it's a matter of hours, ask if he can call another doctor and get you right in. Sure, there is a slim chance he'll call a crony of his and you'll get a rubber-stamp opinion, but most doctors adhere to a strict code of ethics so this isn't likely.

How to find a second doctor

If you haven't been hustled off to the hospital and your doctor tells you you have time to obtain a second opinion, ask him to suggest two or three qualified physicians, then pick one of them. Ask your doctor to have a staff member let the other doctor's office know you will be contacting them.

If you don't wish to see a doctor referred to you by your doctor, follow the strategies presented in Chapter 1 of this book for finding a new doctor. Letting the staff at the doctor's offices you contact know that you aren't looking for a new physician, but simply want a second opinion, may get you in to see a doctor who isn't accepting new patients.

Dealing with records

Have the staff at the second doctor's office contact the first doctor's office for any records they need. While you may have to sign a form allowing this, it is common for these records to be shared in this way. Ask that the copies of the records be transferred prior to your appointment with the second doctor, then follow up to make sure the second doctor's office has received them.

Follow all the strategies we've already covered when you keep your appointment with this doctor, including taking a written list of questions to ask and a notebook in which to record the answers.

The possible outcomes

You may consult another doctor and get the same exact opinion, but that in itself can be comforting. The second doctor may find the same condition, but present you with fresh or different ideas on how to deal with it. Or the second doctor may come to exactly the opposite conclusion as the first doctor. If this is the case, you might ask that the two doctors put their heads together with an eye to finding concert. Another option is to seek a third or even a fourth opinion.

10

The Ubiquitous Paperwork:
Navigating the Records Maze

The doctor entered the room carrying a thick sheaf of papers. Since I had visited him only once I was sure he either had the wrong file or was somehow connected to Homeland Security.

"How did you get that much information about me?" I asked, as he rummaged through the stack.

"You've been here before."

"Once!" I blurted.

"You've seen Dr. Anderson."

The light went on. I had consulted another doctor in the same consortium. The offices were all separate, although geographically close, and each patient had just one file that traveled as needed.

I thought, "This fellow knows more about me than I do." This struck me as funny. I was trying to conceal my laughter when I realized he was bent over the file, chuckling along with me. Apparently I had said it out loud.

This was a great ice breaker and we got along swimmingly.

Record Keeping

Human memory is an unreliable record keeper. No one expects the memory of a fifty-year-old to be as good as that of a twenty-five-year-old. But even a twenty-five-year-old's isn't sufficient for medical record storage. That's why manila folders with colored and numbered tabs were invented.

As you can imagine, your medical record is valuable. It is the tool your doctor uses for managing your health care. For a doctor who sees a large number of patients, it is probably his memory trigger for re-membering who you are when you turn up in his consulting room.

In that folder is the record of what transpired at every office visit you had, dates and treatments, and the results of every completed test, along with documents from other doctors that you may have consulted.

A sign of how valuable your folder is may be seen in how carefully it is guarded—from you. The nurse brings it into the consulting room when she conducts the first part of the interview, but she certainly doesn't let you touch it. When she leaves, she puts it in a holder on the *outside* of the door for the doctor to scoop up when he comes in to talk to you.

Patients frequently wonder, "Well, those are my records, why can't I see them or take them with me?" A logical question. And you do have rights, certainly. You should be able to examine the records and obtain copies of any you want, but the originals belong to your doctor. And, think about it, as a practical matter: Allowing patients to paw through organized files, removing and moving things as they wished would be, well, silly—and possibly dangerous to the patient's health.

If you wish to see your file, just ask.

One way your medical record is valuable is for comparison pur-poses. Noting if something has changed can be vital. This is why stan-dard measurements such as your weight and blood pressure are recorded at nearly every visit.

Things such as film from x-rays taken in your doctor's office are usually stored elsewhere on the premises. Results from tests given at a hospital or an outside laboratory are produced in different forms, de-pending on the machine used to do the test. The digital file, graph, image scan, or film will likely remain in the possession of the institution that produced it. A written report, which tells what the doctor or other expert who read the test has found, will have been sent to your doctor, and a copy of this should be in your file. If your doctor wishes to examine the test results himself, he can request them, or he can go to the hospital or laboratory to do so.

Insurance claims and payment information aren't a part of your medical file; they are retained by your doctor's billing department, whether in-house or out-sourced.

Do ask for any copies you wish. You are entitled to have your records for use in managing your health care. The best time to ask for a copy of the record is at the time it is produced. Going back to retrieve a record is possible, but it is often cumbersome. If you have taken a blood test, for example, ask for a copy of the report at the time you discuss the results with your doctor.

Many doctors and health-care organizations routinely supply the results of a test to the patient in a written form that can be understood by lay people. But if you do not understand, ask that it be explained in terms you can understand. Your comprehension is important so you can make informed decisions.

Another reason to keep copies of your own is as a safeguard against something happening to the originals. For a doctor's office to actually lose a file is almost unheard of, but there is always the risk of human error. Flood, fire, and other natural disasters, as well as acts of terrorism, though unlikely, could happen, rendering useless tons of paper records.

I know of one patient whose whole file was lost by the doctor. He had the good fortune to be a bit of a copy nut and was able to supply his physician with much of what was missing; thus the record was more complete than it might have been.

Having your own copies often helps you to better communicate with your doctor and may save appointment time. Let's say you have recently been experiencing symptoms that make you worry about the health of your heart, and in your personal record, you have copies and dates of previous tests. When you meet with your doctor, you can say something like, "I had an EKG in your office on March 12 that you said was just fine, but I have had some chest pain in the last week. Do you think I should have another?" Since documents are usually arranged in the records folder with the most recent on top, being able to give the doctor the exact date helps him to find it, saving appointment time for other things.

How Records Travel

When more than one doctor is involved in your health care, they will need to share records. Luckily, today it is as easy to send a record across the country as it is across the hall. A fax machine is perfect technology for all paper records, and overnight document services can handle film or other types of material.

However, as simple as it seems, getting a record from one doctor to another sometimes proves to be a monumental task and too often does not get done without some guidance from you.

You need to act as a sort of hall monitor to be sure the required copies move from one place to another as planned. Otherwise you run the risk of spending your appointment time listening as the doctor plays twenty questions with his staff, who finally wind up calling the office of the other doctor and asking for the document to be faxed, only to learn that, for one reason or another, it can't be done right away. You then end up making another appointment to come back when the records have been located and correctly transferred.

When you doctor says something like, "I'll get this to Dr. Smiley," it is easy to believe that this will happen. But doctors are busy, with lots of things on their minds. He may forget by the time he gets to the nurse's station. Or he may verbally pass the request to his assistant who already has both of her hands full of other files.

Here is the procedure for making sure that you and your paperwork arrive for your appointment together:

- Talk to the medical records person in your doctor's office. Ask if she has instructions from the doctor on what to send and where to send it. Request that she include a cover letter explaining why she is sending the records so their arrival isn't a complete mystery to the staff at the other end. This is particularly important if you haven't seen this doctor before because there won't be a file with your name on it awaiting the records.

- When you make the appointment with the second doctor, ask the receptionist if the records have been received. If not, explain that they will be coming. Then call the person you spoke to in your doctor's office and tell her that the records haven't been received yet. Get a commitment from her to send them, or if she already did, that she call the other doctor's staff and clear up the matter.

- At least two business days before your appointment, call to see if the records have been received. If not, contact the medical records person again and get another commitment.

- The following day, call the second doctor's office to see

if the records have arrived. If they haven't, call the medical records person again. (This gives you an opportunity to test the time honored adage that you can catch more flies with honey than you can with vinegar.) Ask that she prepare the paperwork and seal it in an envelope. Tell her you will pick it up and carry it to the second doctor. This call may be the one to get action, saving you a trip to pick up the records, but, if you get another promise, be sure to call the second office to verify that the records did finally make it. If not, pick up the records yourself.

Electronic Record Keeping

The first time your doctor walks into the consulting room with a handheld computer and a stylus instead of your old friend, the manila folder, you may feel as if you had dropped through a trapdoor into the next century. But electronic record keeping is coming to a doctor's office near you. Only an estimated one in five doctors uses the technology as we go to press, but when you consider how quickly Palm Pilots, iPods, and cell phones became commonplace, it may not be long before all records are digitalized.

Inputting a patient's medical records into a computer takes time initially, but it saves time overall. With a little luck, this will lead to more minutes for the doctor to spend with each patient (rather than increasing his patient load with shortened appointment times).

The United States Veterans Administration has been a pioneer in the use of electronic record keeping for its hospitals, clinics, and other facilities. The computer program developed by the VA, called Veterans Health Information and Technology Architecture (VistA), is now available to health-care organizations through a number of service providers. The cost is reduced because VistA is in the public domain and, as such, there are no licensing fees.

VistA and similar systems will provide improved patient care through computerized order entry, bar code medication administration, electronic prescribing, clinical guidelines, and other benefits.

A number of benefits to you as a patient could be accomplished by the use of a computer program. The nurse can enter your vital signs at the time of your appointment. A glance at the screen will tell the doctor if there have been changes. The computer will remind the doctor of any tests or follow-up treatments you need.

The medications you are taking will be on the computer along with any allergies you may have. Some software has been designed to alert the doctor if he enters a new prescription and it conflicts with one you are already taking. Computer printouts eliminate any concern about a pharmacist misreading a doctor's handwriting. If you need a new prescription, the touch of a stylus will print it out at a location outside of the consulting room, where you may get it when you leave the office, or it may be sent directly to the pharmacy to be ready when you arrive to pick it up.

Your paper record can be used by only one person at a time, in one location. An electronic record could be accessed by you in your home, by a hospital getting ready to admit you, and by a surgeon planning his schedule—all at the same time. E-records solve the problem of making copies and faxing or transporting records from one place to another. In an emergency, say while you are on a trip, your records could immediately be consulted by an emergency room doctor.

Even your insurance company, employer, or a government agency may be allowed access to them. Such sharing brings up privacy issues, which are a concern to both doctors and patients. When your records are transferred to an electronic version, ask your doctor about the security of the system he uses, and how he assures that your health records are not available to unauthorized persons.

Keep up with whatever new technology your health-care providers use. The staff will undoubtedly be proud of the system as well as their new skill in using it and will be eager to tell you about it.

Your Personal Health Record (PHR)

Too often, information about our health history is scattered throughout our personal papers or buried in our memories. In either instance pertinent information is often difficult to put our hands on in a moment of need.

Solve this by compiling a personal health record. A PHR will save you so much time that it is well worth the time spent amassing the needed information. A list compiled by the American Health Information Management Association (AHIMA) of what to include in your PHR appears in the Patient's Tool Kit section at the back of this book.

AHIMA is a national, nonprofit, professional association founded in 1928, dedicated to the effective management of the personal health information needed to deliver quality health care to the public. Its 50,000 members are health-care professionals.

A comprehensive set of forms to help you complete your PHR is available from AHIMA at its Web site myPHR.com.

Keep copies of all your test results and other medical records in one folder. Retain one copy of your PHR in this folder and make another one to take with you when you see a doctor.

Having a copy of your PHR with you when you see a doctor for the first time will make filling out the standard clipboard of forms quicker and will assure that you don't forget something important.

A Lifesaving Record

The Vial of Life, or the File of Life, which is the name under which it has been adopted in some communities, offers the opportunity for you to keep a record that may save a life—yours or that of an aging parent or other loved one. Vial of Life is a nonprofit organization sponsored by American Senior Safety Agency, a supplier of medical alarms.

Go to vialoflife.com. Here you will find an emergency medical information form you can fill out on the screen. If you like, you can store the form at the Web site so you can come back and update it as needed. (Vial of Life promises to protect your privacy and not disclose or share any information about you.)

Print three copies of the form. After you print the form, click on the link that says "Print Free Decals." Print out two decals. Put one decal on the front of a plastic freezer bag or an envelope into which you have placed a copy of the form. This bag or envelope goes on the front of your refrigerator, secured with a magnet or tape. If you wish, you may include a picture of the person whose medical record is enclosed. This is particularly useful if there is more than one person in the household. The second decal goes on your front door to alert emergency personnel to look for the form on the refrigerator. Put the second copy of the form in your wallet and the third copy in the glove compartment of your car.

If your community has a drive to popularize this program, emergency personnel will have been briefed to look on the front of the refrigerator if they find a decal on the front door. You might consider starting a program in your community if it hasn't already been done. In the event that a 9-1-1 call is necessary, the written record can save precious minutes. A service club, fire department, police department, or hospital auxiliary, among others, are organizations that might sponsor such a program.

11

Being an Advocate: Talking to the Doctor for Someone Else

It is likely that most communications you have with doctors will concern your own health care. However, there are situations in which you may talk to a doctor on behalf of someone else, perhaps a parent, a spouse, or a friend. Of course the situation can be reversed when you feel the need to have someone beside you, and, if your support in these situations can come from a person you've supported in the past, all the better.

Supporting a friend or relative in this way is often called being a "patient's advocate." But going to the doctor with someone else is not advocacy in the legal sense of the word. That kind of patient advocacy usually deals with privacy or legal issues. These are best handled by a professional advocate or an attorney.

There can be several reasons you might want to offer support. Included among them are:

- Any illness, even a bad cold, can impair a person's ability to speak and listen.

- Hearing loss may interfere with clear communication.

- The side effects of a person's medications may cause an inability to concentrate.

- The power of simple moral support—fears or apprehensions may be alleviated with a familiar companion nearby.

- Shy or easily intimidated people may not ask enough questions or appropriately question the doctor's decisions.
- Many older people may have trouble remembering what the doctor said.

When to offer to step in

Often the person who needs assistance will simply ask when appropriate. Sometimes they won't ask but will jump at the chance if you make the offer. Other times a bit of nudging might be needed.

Suppose you are responsible for one of your parents. Perhaps you have noticed that when you ask your mother what the doctor said, she doesn't remember or she "forgot to ask." Some other clues as to whether a person needs an advocate are statements such as:

- I can never understand what the doctor is saying.

- He has given me a new medicine and I don't know what it's for, but it isn't helping.

- Oh, he told me something about that, but I don't remember.

- I guess I should expect this because I'm getting old.

These are red flags suggesting this person would benefit from your attention as an advocate. Step up to the plate. (If you hear yourself making statements similar to these, it is time for you to acquire some help.)

Dealing with Reluctance

The needs and the feelings of the person for whom you wish to act as an advocate are of foremost importance and must be balanced. Many people wish to retain their independence. Others are simply stubborn and decline any help as a matter of course.

If the person needs an advocate and does not really want one, your task will require careful advance preparation. First be clear in your own mind that this person needs an advocate. Is his hearing impaired? Suffering from failing mental perception? In denial? Forgetful?

Once you are convinced that he is not receiving proper care, use your powers of persuasion to get him to agree to your help. This can be a matter of life and death.

As health problems increase with age, those suffering become more likely to talk about them. In fact, such discussions tend to dominate the conversation at group gatherings as well as in private encounters. Such conversations may allow you an opportunity to show concern and eventually lead to the person's acceptance of you as an advocate.

Be sympathetic, and when you have the opening, offer to go to the doctor with your friend perhaps "just to take notes," so she'll have a record when she gets home.

Another way is to offer to find information for the person or to show him how to do some research for himself. Sometimes this kind of involvement will turn the tide.

Being the Best Advocate You Can Be

Begin by learning everything you can about the problems that sent this person to the doctor in the first place. Information is power. You need to know everything you can find out about her health and the condition for which she is receiving treatment. This includes all of the symptoms she is experiencing and all of the medicine she is taking, prescribed and supplemental. Find out how she feels about the care she has been receiving. Ask if you can view her personal health record if she has one. If she hasn't prepared one, download the forms available at myPHR.com and help her fill them out.

Ask to see all the medicines she's taking. Write their names and dosages down, and check with a pharmacist to see if any conflicts exist. If you find that your friend or relative has a lot of old prescriptions on hand, urge their disposal. That will keep her from using an older prescription by accident or intention. An old prescription might conflict with one issued later or be counterproductive for some other reason.

If she is uneasy about taking someone with her to the doctor because of what she thinks the doctor will say, suggest that she call the office and ask if the doctor minds. Most doctors will welcome such a two-party visit. If you have noticed that your friend or relative needs an advocate, the doctor has probably noticed too.

As a practical matter, it wastes time when a doctor has to repeat himself to a patient who has impaired hearing or understanding, and it is frustrating for a doctor who has given his best advice to find at the next appointment that it has been forgotten or seemingly ignored.

Be wary of a doctor who refuses to allow you to participate without giving you a sound reason.

Prepare for this appointment just like you would for your own appointment. Take two copies of your list of questions so you'll each have one.

If a physical disability or anxiety makes it difficult for a patient to wait a long time in the waiting room, telephone the office, explain the problem, and ask if the doctor is running late. If so, you may want to spend more time waiting at home. You will both be better able to use the

Be Prepared for the Bill

I once witnessed a distressing scene in a doctor's office: A woman and an elderly gentleman were waiting to be called. She asked him about his insurance cards, and he did not seem to have them. She berated him steadily for five minutes. How could he have forgotten them? What did he do with them? She didn't understand *how* he could not have them!

The tirade continued as she had him search his pockets and she ransacked her handbag. She might have been his daughter, his wife, or a caregiver, but she certainly wasn't being helpful. It was distressing.

If your friend or relative carries her own insurance cards, check for them as part of the preparation for the appointment. If her insurance requires a co-pay, be sure she has her checkbook, credit card, or cash to pay it.

appointment time wisely if you are not stressed by a long wait to get in to see the doctor. If possible, try to schedule the appointment early in the day when the doctor is more likely to still be on schedule. Early appointments are also beneficial for an elderly person. Elderly people are likely to be more rested and alert in the morning.

Once you are in the consulting room, you will have to decide how to play your role.

When the doctor walks into the room, watch. Does your friend light up at his presence or does she freeze up? Knowing whether she is comfortable or intimidated will help you guide the communication.

She should have her copy of the questions in hand, but suppose she sits like a statue. Resist the temptation to take over. Address your remarks to her: "Beth, were you going to ask the doctor about your leg cramps?"

Keep prompting as necessary. With luck it will be like getting the first olive out of the bottle—the rest will pour out. If a question arises in your mind that she does not ask, ask it of her.

"Beth, do you think you should ask about the swelling in your ankles?" This will give her the chance to put the question in her own words and to add to it if necessary.

A word of caution: When acting as a patient advocate for elderly patients, be alert for a doctor who blames problems on "natural aging." Most conditions now can be treated and cured even in very old people.

Take notes. Go over these notes together after the appointment.

Nursing Homes

If you are helping someone who is in an assisted-living facility or a nursing home, you will need to learn how medical attention is handled for the residents. Some facilities have an in-house physician who comes at regular intervals to see patients and write prescriptions.

A nursing home may employ a doctor to act as medical director. This doctor may visit on a regular schedule seeing only the residents who need him. Nurses monitor patient condition and medication the rest of the time. In this case, you will want to communicate with the nurses on a regular basis and arrange to be present at the time of the medical director's visit if you need to speak with him.

A periodic check of meds is also prudent if a person is in a nursing home. It is more difficult for you to keep current under those circumstances, since a doctor can prescribe without your immediate knowledge.

Some institutions provide transportation so that patients may see their own doctors. Sometimes they select one day each week as "doctor day." Residents need to make their appointments accordingly. Be sure that both your friend or relative and the doctor understand this.

Spouses

"My husband won't go to the doctor," is a wail that appears in advice columns regularly.

Some day, researchers may discover why so many men are reluctant to go to the doctor. It may be macho feelings, worry about appearing weak, the conviction that if he ignores the problem it will go away, or just plain fear. Whatever the reason, the fact remains that men resist going to the doctor more than women.

The tendency of men to avoid seeking medical attention is attracting national attention. An article in an *AARP Bulletin* noted that this tendency is fueling a silent health crisis. The article points out men have a one-in-two lifetime chance of developing cancer, compared with a one-in-three chance for women. Also men typically die about five years earlier than women.

For wives trying to encourage husbands to go to the doctor, help is available from The Men's Health Network (MHN). This nonprofit organization has as one of its goals "to encourage women to expand on their traditional role as the family's health-care provider and activist for the enhancement of health-care services."

As a wife, try to interest your husband in the Web site at menshealthnetwork.org as a way of showing him you aren't the only person who thinks he should go to the doctor. For example, the MHN quotes a survey that shows that 70 percent of men over fifty change their daily routines to accommodate frequent bathroom trips, rather than seek medical attention.

As the birthdays keep coming and health problems are more at the forefront of both your lives, it may be prudent to go to the doctor with your spouse.

How do you decide when it is the right thing to do? Watch for the same things that you watch for in an elderly parent—failing eyesight or hearing, any signs of confusion. Your spouse can probably manage alone if the appointment is for a sore throat, but if the sore throat has persisted for more than two weeks, plan to go along. You know your spouse and his or her symptoms better than anyone other than your spouse. If he or she will not ask searching questions of the doctor, is inclined to stick to preconceived notions about the condition, or is likely to minimize the diagnosis, you need to be present.

If you are keeping an appointment together, you will get the most out of your time by settling any differences that you have first. The doctor's office is not a battleground. He is not a referee. Just because there are two of you doesn't mean you'll get double time. As always, decide what questions you need answered and write them down. Make a copy for each of you. Decide who is going to ask them. One of you should act as the note taker. If you plan before the appointment, you will have plenty of time to get the information you need.

Doctors used to ask a spouse to step out of the consulting room if they were going to perform any examination that required touching. Out with the spouse, in with the nurse, was the rule, and it may be what you remember. Not all doctors follow that procedure today. If you think that such an exam might take place, decide ahead of time how you will handle it. If you think you will be embarrassed or squeamish, leave. You can come back. The doctor will understand.

Your Official Standing

When you go to the doctor with a friend, parent or spouse who is capable of acting for herself, you will not need any paperwork. If you must act for someone who is not able to act for herself, you will save time by establishing your legal position.

A durable power of attorney for health care, sometimes called a health-care proxy, is a document that names someone to act for the person who signs it. It enables that one person to make decisions about health care for another if that person is unable to make them. As you can imagine, it behooves you to have this form filled out and signed before a problem arises.

Preprinted forms are available, but it may be better if it is prepared with help from an attorney, especially if you wish to spell out additional provisions such as organ donation. Alternate agents to act for the patient, in the event the first person isn't available, may be listed. The original should be kept on file by the patient, with a copy given to the other parties and a copy placed in the files of the primary-care physician.

The durable power of attorney for health care may spell out your rights to the medical records of the signer. But in the matter of medical records, a piece of federal legislation has come into play: the Health Insurance Portability and Accountability Act (HIPAA), and under that act, the Standards for Privacy of Individually Identifiable Health Information. It is this portion of the act that has most affected the individual patient. It produced another piece of paper that a patient needs to sign authorizing the release of records to one or more persons. You may have signed one yourself and filed it with your own doctor when the act took effect. The person for whom you are acting will need to sign a release naming you as one entitled to receive his or her medical records. Otherwise you will not be able to get a copy of procedures or test results, even for file purposes.

In the way of government regulations, although this act was designed to reduce paperwork, it has not yet done so. The act is extensive. Complete information is available at hipaa.org.

Living Wills

It is hard to think of yourself as unconscious, unable to communicate or recognize your loved ones, or in a state of complete dependence on others. But it could happen, and even if you have talked about your preferences for care with the people closest to you, if you do not have a living will or a power of attorney for health care, there won't be much those people can do.

Laws vary from one jurisdiction to another, so your best bet is to request a form for a living will from the health department of the state in which you live. Wherever that may be, the basic procedure is the same: You will fill out the form, sign it, get it witnessed, and distribute copies to family members, your doctor, your lawyer, and your own medical file. You will be considering what quality of life means to you and what treatments you would want to have or not have if you are not able to make those decisions when they need to be made. It is important to remember that you can change or cancel your living will at any time, but that it cannot be overridden or changed by anyone else.

There is a sample living will in the Patient's Tool Kit that follows.

Patient's Tool Kit

Doctor Rating Chart

Photocopy and use the chart below for each health-care professional you are rating. A rating of 5 is highest, 1 is lowest.

Name:

	1	2	3	4	5
Listens attentively					
Appears interested					
Seems compassionate					
Makes me feel at ease					
Has a sense of humor					
Disciplinary actions pending					
Training					

Personal observations:

List of Medications

Photocopy the form below. List your prescriptions and supplements and how much and how often you take them. When folded in half, the form is the size of a credit card and will fit in your wallet. Keep it with you. Be sure to update it when your medicines change.

·
·
·

Name_____		
Medication	Mg	Dosage

·
·
·

(Fold here.)

Prescription Checklist

If your doctor is prescribing a medication you should do all of the following:

- Write down the name of the medication.

- Ask what the goal of prescribing it is. Will it effect a cure or simply alleviate symptoms?

- Ask about alternative medications and how they differ.

- Ask what the likely consequences of not taking it are.

- Ask how long it will take to start working.

- Find out what side effects, if any, may result from taking it. If there are side effects, ask what you can do to alleviate them.

- Ask if the generic equivalent is acceptable. This is important because generics usually cost substantially less than their brand-name counterparts. Many insurance policies pay a larger portion of the cost of a generic drug to encourage cost savings. Often a generic drug is okay, but your doctor may feel a certain brand-name drug is superior to its generic equivalent.

- Write down how your medicine is to be taken, at what dosage and at what intervals. Both of these things will be on the prescription label, but this gives you a chance to double check the pharmacy's accuracy.

- Ask if there are any special instructions such as whether it should be taken with food or an hour before bedtime.

- Call to your doctor's attention the list of medicines and supplements you are already taking, and ask if there is any conflict among them.

- Ask if you can stop taking the medication when you

begin to feel better or, as is the case with most antibiotics, if you finish the whole prescription even if you feel well? Some medications require that you wean yourself off them by taking diminishing doses. Of course, some you'll be on for the rest of your life or until another alternative comes along.

- Ask if the prescription is refillable without another office visit.

Your pharmacist is qualified to help you with these questions if you don't get them answered to your satisfaction by your doctor.

Six Things You Can Do to Conquer Your Medical Fears

What if you are just plain scared? It can happen to anyone. Here are some strategies to help you conquer your fears:

1) Learn all you can. You will find that a good deal of the fear factor is removed if you have gained knowledge about your condition and its possibilities and probabilities. Knowledge is power. And knowledge will give you power to deal with your predicament.

2) Examine other fears in your life and figure out how you managed them. Maybe you are afraid of heights, afraid of flying, or afraid of dogs. Will any of the strategies you have developed for coping with those fears work? (If it takes a couple of Bloody Marys to get you on a plane, you had better find another way to get to your appointment unafraid.)

3) Talk to God. Prayer works well for those who believe in it, as does asking others to pray for you or with you. There have been several patient studies indicating that those who have someone praying for them do better than those who do not.

4) Write down exactly why you are afraid. Fears set down in black and white lose their nebulous monster-under-the-bed power. They become something you can confront, not something floating on the fringes of your mind making you anxious.

5) Bag the guilt. Guilt can add to your fear. "Did I see the doctor soon enough? Should I have made this appointment months ago? Did I continue to take a medication that has come under suspicion? Is my problem my fault?" It is human nature to want to blame someone when something goes wrong. If you can't find anyone else, you'll blame yourself.

Yes, you may have been doing something unhealthy. It seems one lifestyle choice or another comes under fire every day. No one has a crystal ball. Even if you were doing something unhealthy, don't play the blame game. It is a waste of time and energy.

Of course, quit any unhealthy behaviors and concentrate on what you can do to prepare for what may lie ahead and what you can do to get well.

6)   Confess your fears to someone you trust. Often, when you state your fears aloud, they sound minor and silly. Another person can help just by listening, but he or she may also be able to help you put them in perspective.

Don't go to someone who isn't a good listener or plays the "I can top that" game. If you can find someone who has gone through the same experience, that person may be your best source of comfort.

Prescription Problems and Possible Solutions

Problem	**Possible Solutions**
Impaired vision	• Ask pharmacist to use large print on label. • Use a magnifying glass to check labels before taking medications.
Impaired hearing	• Let others know if you did not hear the instructions. • Ask doctor/pharmacist to write instructions. • Ask someone to go with you to the doctor.
Complex dosage schedule	• Write down your schedule clearly and use color to differentiate times of day. Use daily/weekly medication dispensers. Coordinate the time to take medication with specific activities (e.g., meal time, time of favorite television program, when mail arrives, etc.).
Forgetfulness	• Use memory aids and daily or weekly medication dispensers. • Place notes to yourself where you will see them.
Limited mobility	• Use a pharmacy that will deliver prescriptions (cost may be higher).
Limited use of hands	• Ask pharmacist for easy-to-open bottle caps.
Multiple medications	• Have doctor evaluate medication

	regimen regularly.
	• Use a pharmacy that keeps a patient profile for customers.
Multiple doctors	• Make sure each doctor knows all medications you are taking.
	• Purchase all prescriptions at only one pharmacy.
Cost of medications	• Call local pharmacies and compare prices.
	• Ask doctor or pharmacist whether a generic drug will be as effective and less costly.
	• Ask doctor or pharmacist if you qualify for a patient assistance program through a drug company.

Questions to Ask if Your
Doctor Wants to Order Tests

- What will this test tell us?

- Will it confirm a diagnosis or rule something out, or is it meant to measure the severity of a problem?

- How will the results of this test impact our decisions on future treatment?

- Are there risks associated with this test?

- Is this test invasive? If so, in what way?

- How long will the test take?

- What pretest preparation, such as fasting, is required?

- Where will the test be administered?

- Will anesthesia be needed?

- If so, will it be local or general?

- Will the test require hospitalization?

- Will I need to schedule someone to drive me home?

- Who will read and interpret the test results?

- How long will it take to get the results?

- How will I be notified of the results?

- How much does this test cost?

- Is the test experimental?

- Are there other tests that should be considered in lieu of this one?

- If so, what are the differences and merits of each?

- If I decide not to have the test, what are my other options?

How to Create a One-page Medical History

Allow:

- One paragraph for name, date of birth, height, weight, marital status, work status, and exercise program.

- One paragraph for childhood diseases and immunizations.

- One paragraph for surgeries, including dates and complications.

- One paragraph for serious illnesses, treatments, and any persistent symptoms.

- One paragraph for any medications that have not agreed with you. Attach a copy of your list of medications.

- One paragraph listing your family health history. Include the major diseases that have afflicted close relatives.

- One paragraph concerning your regular health care and treatments you currently receive.

- A sentence concerning your use of alcohol, tobacco, and other addictive substances.

- Take this one-page medical history when you are seeing a new doctor for the first time.

How to Create a
Personal Health Record (PHR)

A personal health record (PHR) is a collection of important information, that you actively maintain and update, about your health or the health of someone you're caring for, such as a parent or a child.

When collecting information from your health records, be sure to include:

- Personal identification, including name, birth date, and social security number

- People to contact in case of emergency: Names, addresses, and phone numbers of your physician, dentist, and other specialists

- Health insurance information

- Living wills and advance directives

- Organ donor authorization

- A list with dates of significant illnesses and surgeries

- Current medications and dosages

- Immunizations and their dates

- Allergies

- Important events, dates, and hereditary conditions in your family history

- Most recent physical examination

- Opinions of specialists

- Important tests results

- Eye and dental records

- Correspondence between you and your health provider(s)

- Permission forms for release of information, operations,

and other medical procedures

- Any information you want to include about your health—your exercise regimen, any herbal supplements you take, and any counseling you receive.

This list was compiled by The American Health Information Management Association. AHIMA is a national, nonprofit, professional association, founded in 1928, dedicated to the effective management of personal health information needed to deliver quality health care to the public. Find more about AHIMA at www.myphr.com.

Advocate's To-Do List

If you are acting as a patient advocate for a friend or relative, the list below gives you a place to start. Each situation is different. You may not feel comfortable doing some things on the list and you may wish to add others.

- Make or confirm appointments.

- Discuss with your friend or relative what the goals of the appointment are.

- Help the person write out questions to ask the doctor at each visit.

- Take to the appointment a list of medications being taken by the friend or relative. Include any supplements, such as St. John's wort.

- Take notes at the appointment.

- Be sure the friend or relative takes any necessary insurance cards to the appointment and that he or she has a checkbook or other way to pay any co-payments due at that time.

- Determine if the person has been following the doctor's orders.

- Research this person's illnesses or complaints on the Internet.

- Take a current list of the person's medications to a pharmacist and ask that he review it for conflicts.

- Help make decisions on health-care matters such as the need for inpatient procedures or hospitalization.

- Help the person to compile a personal health history (PHR).

- Help this person obtain a durable power of attorney for health-care.

- Help prepare a living will.

A Sample Living Will

My Living Will

I, _____ , willfully and voluntarily make known my desire that my dying not be artificially prolonged under the circumstances set forth below. It is my intention and hope that this declaration be honored by my family and physician as the final expression of my right to refuse medical intervention. ACCORDINGLY, IF AT ANY TIME

- I have a terminal condition—including a coma or persistent vegetative state,

AND

- my attending physician determines that my condition is irreversible—that is, I will not recover no matter what medical interventions are provided,

AND

- I am unable to give directions regarding my medical care,

THEN I direct that all medical interventions be withheld or withdrawn except for those interventions necessary to provide me with comfort care and to alleviate pain. ADDITIONALLY (check either *a* or *b* below),

a. _____ I DO NOT want food, water, or other nourishment or fluids provided to me through tubes placed in my veins, nose, throat, or surgically placed in my stomach when the above conditions are met and I am unable to eat or drink by myself.

OR

b. ____ I DO want food, water, or other nourishment or fluids provided to me through tubes placed in my veins, nose, throat, or surgically placed in my stomach when the above conditions are met and I am unable to eat or drink by myself.

Finally, I have written below other instructions or limitations associated with my care for when I have a terminal, irreversible condition and I cannot make decisions for myself.

_____

_____

_____

_____

_____

_____

(If none, write "NONE")

Separate from what I have indicated above (check either *a* or *b* below),

a. ___ I DO want to be an organ/tissue donor after I die. If I choose to be a donor, I grant permission for artificial support to be maintained only for that period of time required to ensure the viability and removal of such organs/tissue.

OR

b. ____ I DO NOT want to be an organ/tissue donor.

I understand and accept the consequences of the directives I have indicated above. I also understand that as long as I am capable of making decisions for myself, I can revoke this Living Will at any time.

Signed: _____ Date: _____

Witnesses' Statement

We believe that the person who has completed this Living Will understands the meaning of what has been indicated herein. We also believe that this Living Will has been completed freely and in good faith. We are not members of this person's family, nor will we benefit financially from this person's death. Finally, we are not this person's physician or employees of the physician, hospital, or other health-care facility from which this person receives care.

Name: _____

Signature: _____ Date: _____

Name: _____

Signature: _____ Date: _____

This sample living will is not to replace legal advice from a qualified attorney. Consult your legal advisor.

Web Sites of Interest

mayoclinic.com *(Mayo Clinic's web site)*

cdc.gov *(Center for Disease Control)*

healthfinder.gov *(Developed by the United States Department of Health and Human Services, information from over 1,500 agencies, organizations, and universities.)*

nihseniorhealth.gov *(This site also provides audio.)*

niapublications.org *(National Institute on Aging)*

nih.gov *(National Institute of Health for A to Z medical information)*

nlm.nih.gov *(National Library of Medicine for current medical news and a link to Medline where you can have information for a specific problem sent to you free by e-mail)*

unitedhealthfoundation.org *(For information on how your state ranks among others for health care, and health tips you can use.)*

patientsarepowerful.org *(For steps to patient empowerment.)*

talkaboutrx.org *(National Council on Patient Education and Information for extensive information relating to prescriptions)*

MDVIP.com *(For information on "boutique" medicine.)*

myphr.com *(Free health forms and information on setting up and keeping your health information stored on line.)*

ahima.org *(American Health Information Management Association)*

seniorsafety.com *(For link to the Vial of Life website and extensive information on medical alerts and alarms to insure your safety.)*

menshealth.com *(Provides daily tips and information on men's health issues.)*
Ratemds.com *(Patients rate their doctors.)*

Also look for links to the following. (You can use your new searching or "Googling" skills.)

AARP Health Care

Alzheimers Association

American Medical Association

Citizens' Council on Health Care

Department of Health and Human Services

   • My Family Health Portrait

DrKoop.com

Electronic Privacy Information Center

healthfinder®

Harris Interactive® Healthcare News

Health Hippo

Healthy People 2010

Health Privacy Project

Institute for Healthcare Advancement

KidsHealth

Medicare

My Health eVet

MyHealthTestReminder.com

Office of Civil Rights

   • Fact Sheet: Privacy and Your Health Information

   • Fact Sheet: Your Health Information Privacy Rights

PrivacyExchange

Put It in Writing

Save the Patient

Social Security

Suggested Reading

The Intelligent Patient's Guide to The Doctor-Patient Relationship: Learning How to Talk So Your Doctor Will Listen. Barbara M. Korsch, M.D., Caroline Harding, 1997, published by Oxford University Press.

The Savvy Patient: How to be an Active Participant in Your Medical Care. David R. Stutz, M.D.; Bernard Feder; and the editors of Consumer Reports Books, 1990, published by Consumer Reports Books.

The American Medical Association Guide to Talking to Your Doctor. Angela Perry, M.D., 2001, published by John Wiley and Sons Inc.

The Patient's Guide to Medical Tests, 2d ed.: Everything You Need to Know about the Tests Your Doctor Orders. Joseph C. Segen, M.D., F.C.A.P., F.A.S.C.P. and Josie Wade, R.N., 2002, published by Facts on File.

Dr. Ruth's Sex After 50: Revving up the Romance, the Passion and the Excitement. Dr. Ruth K. Westheimer, 2005, published by Quill Driver Books.

Live Longer, Live Better. Peter H. Gott, M.D., 2004, published by Quill Driver Books.

It's Never Too Late to Be Happy! Muriel James, Ed.D., 2002, published by Quill Driver Books.

The Memory Manual: Ten Simple Things You Can Do to Improve Your Memory After 50. Betty Fielding, 1999, published by Quill Driver Books.

Could It Be B$_{12}$?: An Epidemic of Misdiagnoses. Sally M. Pacholok, R.N., Jeffrey J. Stuart, D.O., 2005, published by Quill Driver Books.

AARP The Magazine, published bimonthly by The American Association of Retired Persons, and the *AARP Bulletin*. Both the magazine and the bulletin are a benefit included in AARP membership. The web address is aarp.org.

Index

Physician 12
National Institute on Aging 2
National Institutes of Health 44, 47, 66
natural remedies 13
naturopathic and homeopathic medicine
  13
naturopathic.com 13
Navane (thiothixene) 51
Neurological surgery 71
neurology 71
New England Journal of Medicine, The
  44, 53
nih.gov 66
Northwestern University Center for
  Clinical Resear 44
Norvasc (amiodipine besylate) 51
Nuclear medicine 71
nurse 29, 30, 39, 77, 91, 93
nurse practitioner 11, 12
nursing home 91
nutrition 33

O

obesity 5
obstetrics and gynecology 71
oncologist 34
ophthalmologist 37
ophthalmology 71
organ donation 93
orthopaedic surgery 71
osteopathic.org 4
osteoporosis 62
Ostomy Association 23
otolaryngology 71
overmedication 49
oxygen 60

P

Pacholok, Sally M. 24
pain control 75
palpation 31
pap test 64
pathology 71
patient/surgeon relationship 71
patient's advocate 87
Patients Bill of Rights 76
pediatrics 71
penicillin 50
personal health record (PHR) 17, 85,
  89
personal medical history 32
pharmaceuticals 13, 52
pharmacies, Canadian 56
pharmacies, Mexican 57

pharmacist 3, 51, 54, 99
pharmacy 51, 52, 55, 57, 85
pharmicist 89
Phoenix, Arizona 3
Phoenix Magazine 3
PHR 85
physical examination 59
physical medicine and rehabilitation 71
physical therapy 32
physician assistant (PA) 12
physician's assistant 9
plastic surgery 71
platelets 61
polyps 64
power of attorney 76, 93, 94
prayer 25
pre-op appointment 74, 75
prescriptions 6, 9, 27, 32, 49, 51, 53,
  54, 57, 75, 85
preventive medicine 71
primary-care physician 1, 2, 3, 4, 7, 32,
  34, 35, 39, 50, 53, 69, 70, 93
privacy issues 85
privacy statement 76
prostate-specific antigen (PSA) 63
psychiatry 71
pulmonary function tests (PFT) 63
pulmonary specialist 35

R

radiation 62, 68
radioactive tracer 62, 65
radiologist 60, 67
radiology 71
Ratemds.com 10
receptionist 38, 39
record keeping, electronic 84
recovery plan 73
recovery room 77
rectum 64
red blood cells 61
refill prescriptions 55, 75
retainer medicine 13
risks 65
R$_x$ 54

S

samples 52
scanning camera 62
scoliosis 37
search engines 43, 47
second opinion 78
seizures 64
small intestine 61

About the Author

Patricia A. Agnew is a resident of Lake Havasu City, Arizona. A graduate of the College of Journalism at the University of Nebraska, she has been a reporter and columnist for newspapers in Nebraska and a writer for the *Denver Post* in Denver, Colorado. Her articles have appeared in a number of Denver area magazines, *Southwest Art*, and *Writer's Digest Yearbook*. She has written features for the Web site of Environment News Service. In addition to writing, she worked as an investigative assistant in the sheriff's office of Grand County, Colorado. She is a thirty-two-year member and past president of the Denver Women's Press Club; a member of the Society of Southwest Authors, Tucson, Arizona; and a thirty-year member of Colorado Press Women. She is married and has three daughters.

Other Great Titles from Quill Driver Books

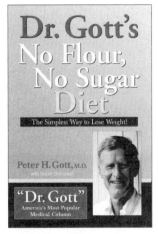
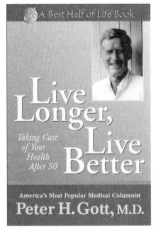

Other Great Books in

The Best Half of Life® Series

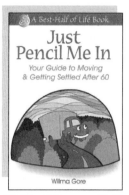

Just Pencil Me In
Your Guide to Moving & Getting Settled After 60

by Willma Willis Gore

The first book to address the unique, distinct concerns encountered by those of us over 60 when faced with relocating. Crammed with indispensable tips to make your move uncomplicated and enjoyable.

$12.95 • 176 pages • 6"x9"
Index • Bibliography
Resources section

Videotape Your Memoirs
The Perfect Way to Preserve Your Family's History
by Suzanne Kita and Harriet Kinghorn

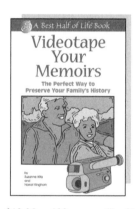

Learn how to videotape your life story; the best and easiest way to record your memoirs. This is the first book of it's kind!

$12.95 • 128 pages • 6" x 9"
Index • Bibliography

The Memory Manual
10 Simple Things You Can Do to Improve Your Memory After *50*
By Betty Fielding

No gimmicks, no long codes or systems to study and memorize, just a simple, holistic program that will get you or a loved one on track to a better memory and a fuller life!

$14.95 • 6" x 9" • 212 pages
Bibliography • Index • Resources